Focal Therapy of Prostate Cancer

Stefan Thüroff • Christian G. Chaussy

Editors

Focal Therapy of Prostate Cancer

An Emerging Strategy for Minimally
Invasive, Staged Treatment

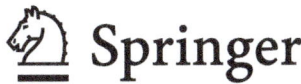 Springer

Editors
Stefan Thüroff
Department of Urology
Klinikum München-Harlaching
München
Germany

Christian G. Chaussy
Department of Urology
University of Regensburg Caritas Hospital
St. Josef
Regensburg
Germany

ISBN 978-3-319-14159-6   ISBN 978-3-319-14160-2   (eBook)
DOI 10.1007/978-3-319-14160-2

Library of Congress Control Number: 2015935191

Springer Cham Heidelberg New York Dordrecht London

Printed on acid-free paper

Springer is part of Springer Science+Business Media (www.springer.com)

Preface

Over the past 25 years, the average life expectancy for men has increased by almost 4 years, and the age at prostate cancer detection has decreased by an average of 10 years, with diagnosis being increasingly at early stages where curative therapy is still possible. These changing trends in the age and extent of malignancy at diagnosis have revealed limitations in conventional curative therapies for prostate cancer. This is a significant risk of aggressive cancer recurrence and a risk of long-term genitourinary morbidity and a detrimental impact on patient quality of life (QOL). In some cases, radical prostatectomy can be considered an overtreatment. Though this approach offers superior oncological control, the majority of men will risk lifestyle-altering side effects and will find the outcome bothersome. Greater awareness of the shortcomings in radical prostatectomy, external radiotherapy, and brachytherapy has prompted the search for alternative curative as well as cytoreductive palliative therapies that offer comparable rates of cancer control and less treatment-related morbidity to better preserve QOL.

The least invasive "therapy" of the prostate cancer (PCa) treatment spectrum is active surveillance, which defers treatment until PSA or biopsy indicate progression. The rational of active surveillance for low-risk, low-stage prostate cancer is sound; however, undertreatment is an inherent risk of active surveillance. In many cases, however, active surveillance is poorly adhered to by patients and physicians, and many seek radical treatment. This can be the result of feeling uncomfortable with the idea of leaving a curable cancer untreated and possibly missing the opportunity of cure. Nearly ¼–⅓ of patients leave the "active surveillance" concept because the "do nothing" approach carries the psychological burden of allowing a known cancer to affect their QOL.

This opens the possibility of noninvasive prostate cancer therapies like focal therapy. Although this approach is new for PCa, focal therapy is used extensively for other diseases, for instance, lumpectomy for breast cancer and cryotherapy for cervical carcinoma. Focal therapy for PCa is a management concept whereby active therapy is delivered to malignant portions of the gland, eradicating exclusively the known and targeted cancer while sparing unaffected tissue and reducing the morbidity of treatment. It combines active treatment of the identified clinical significant disease with active surveillance of the remaining unaffected tissue and offers an intermediate means of active management of PCa with potentially better preserved QOL for the patient.

There is hope that focal therapy for the treatment of PCa will maintain curative and survival rates comparable to those of conventional primary surgical and radiation therapy.

In this book, we present new and promising diagnostics, stress the reason and arguments for the recent evolution of this new concept of focal prostate cancer therapy, and present the potential application of this management approach within a spectrum of therapeutic options currently available for patients with localized PCa.

Regensburg, Germany   Christian G. Chaussy
München, Germany   Stefan Thüroff

Contents

Part III   New Therapeutic Options for Focal Therapy of PCa

Part I

Background

What Will Happen If I Do Nothing? Natural Development of Prostate Cancer Under Consideration of Histopathological Patterns

1

Glen Kristiansen

Contents

1.1 Introduction

The marked discrepancy of a high prostate cancer incidence and a comparatively low mortality we observe in the USA and the western world constitutes the core problem of clinicians and patients alike in the handling of newly diagnosed prostate cancer cases [1]. Although termed "cancer", which evokes images of a life-threatening and devastating disease, its clinical courses may be highly variable, and a large fraction of patients will not succumb to it but die of other causes. This notion of prostate cancer as a "pet" version of cancer has long predominated, and into the late 1980s, it was a common approach, especially in Scandinavian countries but also in the UK, to spare patients active therapy in favour of watchful waiting. However, a few cases exhibited more aggressive courses that did indeed follow the widely assumed carnivore nature

G. Kristiansen, MD
Institute of Pathology, University Hospital of Bonn (UKB),
Sigmund-Freud-Strasse 25, Bonn 53127, Germany
e-mail: Glen.Kristiansen@ukb.uni-bonn.de

© Springer International Publishing Switzerland 2015
S. Thüroff, C.G. Chaussy (eds.), *Focal Therapy of Prostate Cancer:
An Emerging Strategy for Minimally Invasive, Staged Treatment*,
DOI 10.1007/978-3-319-14160-2_1

cancer is ascribed in general. The introduction of serum PSA testing and prolonged life expectancy we faced in recent decades further contributed to the gradually rising awareness that prostate cancer may not only be a common age-related ailment that one dies with, but a potentially life-shortening disease worth treating that is more prevalent than thought before. These developments have induced our interest in the natural course of this disease, to better understand whom to treat at all and how to stratify optimal therapeutic options. These are recurring questions of newly diagnosed prostate cancer patients: Will I die from cancer? Will I need treatment? What are the options? Since all therapeutic options imply a certain degree of morbidity that may seriously impair the quality of life (e.g. impotence, incontinence, etc.), the increasingly enlightened patient will finally ask: And what would happen if I did nothing? Given the fact of a still ongoing discussion of the principal validity of the term "cancer" for well-differentiated tumours (Gleason score 6) among experts, this must be even more puzzling to patients [2]. More recently, the validity of primary diagnostics has been questioned, and this point may indeed have escaped a wider recognition in patient circles for a longer time. Among experts it was always evident that prostate biopsy diagnostics provides merely an approximation towards the full extent of prostate cancer (as seen in radical prostatectomy specimens) and necessarily suffers on the one hand from sampling bias during the biopsy and on the other hand from interpretation bias or interobserver variability in the histological analysis. So finally, we also have to answer the patient's question on the correctness of his biopsy result. Therefore, this chapter aims to provide a summary of our current understanding of prostate cancer behaviour and the validity of our contemporary biopsy-based histological diagnostics.

1.2 Epidemiology

In western countries, prostate cancer is a common disease among ageing men [1]. Autopsy series have consistently demonstrated that a considerable proportion of men harbour microscopically detectable foci of prostatic adenocarcinoma with increasing rates with age. The study of Gaynor et al. found a carcinoma incidence of 18.4 % at autopsy in total, approaching 40 % in patients over 80 years [3]. This is in good concordance with other studies. Breslow et al. described a cancer prevalence rate of 30 % in patients >70 years, again with a strong age dependency but also geographical variations, i.e. particularly high rates in Sweden and Jamaica and lower rates in Israel and Singapore [4]. Sakr et al. reported an incidence of invasive carcinoma in 64 % of patients over 70 [5]. Even the early reports unite in the notion that the rates of detected carcinoma widely exceed the rate of carcinomas that had clinically become evident before. The term *latent prostate carcinoma* has been coined for these neoplasms that represent incidental findings at autopsy and that did apparently not shorten the patient's life span. It builds also the foundation of the widespread appreciation of prostate cancer being most commonly a harmless and insignificant cancer of older men, whereas only a minority suffers and succumbs to a lethal version of this disease. Only recently it has been demonstrated that even these latent cancers may indeed exhibit features of aggressive disease. Gleason scores of 7 or higher were found in 31.6 % and this percentage even increases with age [6]. Since the widespread application of PSA testing in western countries introduces a detection bias, this contemporary autopsy study from non-screened countries is particularly valuable. All these studies corroborate age as a major risk factor for the diagnosis of prostate cancer, which constitutes an increasing economical problem in ageing societies.

1.3 The Natural Course of Prostate Cancer

The historical pathology textbook from E. Kaufmann (1911) stated on the subject of prostate cancer, "Of particular importance is carcinoma of the prostate. Grossly, the discrimination from hyperplasia can often be difficult, particularly since it has only a limited tendency to invade its vicinity and it also displays little decay. Some carcinomas are so small, that they can be overlooked; wasting and bone metastases may then be the primary symptoms" [7]. Although a bit brief, these historical sentences describe a few characteristic features of prostate cancer that have not lost their validity. In the pre-biopsy era of Kaufmann's statement, prostate cancer was often not diagnosed until (too) late, since early symptoms are lacking. The correct diagnosis was made, if at all, at autopsy, demonstrating extensive "ostitis carcinomatosa". We know now that once prostate cancer is progressing from an organ-confined to a more extensive disease, it first spreads to local lymph nodes (which thus are sampled surgically) and later shows an unparalleled propensity for bone metastases, usually affecting the lumbar spine first and other bones in due course. The final step is further systemic spread with metastases to parenchymal organs, heralding tumour-associated death. However, the individual natural course of prostate cancer is highly variable, showing marked differences that render an individual prognostic estimation difficult.

1.4 What Can We Learn from Watchful Waiting Cohorts?

Several studies have investigated the clinical course of prostate cancer that has been treated conservatively after its diagnosis. Chodack et al. provided an early meta-analysis of six nonrandomised studies from different countries (Israel, Scotland, USA and Sweden), encompassing 828 patients with a median age of 69 years and a median follow-up time of 6.5 years. As expected, tumour grade and patient age were identified as prognostic parameters for tumour-associated mortality. After 10 years of follow-up, only 5.8 % of grade 1 patients, 6.4 % of grade 2 patients but 41.9 % of grade 3 patients had died from prostate cancer. The authors therefore concluded that prostate cancer is a progressive disease, when conservatively managed, but also that watchful waiting was an eligible therapeutic strategy for patients with grade 1 or 2 tumours, particularly if their life expectancy is below 10 years. Although this appears plausible, we have to bear in mind some biases in the study design. Firstly, a central review of histology or cytology was not conducted; secondly, the WHO grading applied here is not used anymore; and thirdly, even patients that eventually received either local or systemic tumour therapy were kept in the study [8].

Albertsen et al. provided a retrospective population-based study of either observed or conservatively treated prostate cancer patients with a long-term follow-up median of 24 years [9]. The cohort consisted of 767 men who were diagnosed between 1971 and 1984. The majority of cases were diagnosed by transurethral resections (60 %) or needle biopsies (26 %), but also cases with "simple open prostatectomy" were enclosed. Age at diagnosis was 69 years and significant comorbidity was reported. A central review of Gleason scores ensured comparable histologic parameters. The results of this often-cited study provide a detailed description of outcomes according to patient age and Gleason scores. The data illustrates impressively that cancer-specific mortality increases with Gleason scores, which is particular relevant to younger men, whereas with increasing patient age, the overall mortality becomes a confounding factor. This study, which is a sequel [10], also demonstrates that after 15 years of follow-up, the data does not change markedly anymore. The prognosis of low-grade tumours (Gleason scores 2–6) is relatively good, as the tumour-specific survival rate of 70 % of patients >70 years with Gleason 6 cases shows. This changes abruptly with tumours of Gleason scores of 7 or higher, and this effect is pronounced in younger men and is ameliorated by age. Although this study is only younger than a decade, it is difficult to translate its results into current practice. First, these results from the pre-PSA era may not be immediately transferable to PSA-screened patients. Second, the initial diagnostic workup is inhomogeneous and is not comparable to modern needle biopsy regimens. The same holds true for Gleason scoring, which rarely shows scores below 6 in contemporary practice; possibly a second round of central review could resolve this matter. Third, there is a mild contamination by patients treated with prostatectomy, which is not a strictly conservative approach.

Cuzick et al. also analysed a conservatively treated prostate cancer cohort but involved not only histological (Gleason) grade but also tumour stage and serum PSA as potential prognostic parameters [11]. The cohort consisted of 2,333 men with a median age of 70 years, of which 1,663 were left untreated and 670 patients received early anti-hormonal therapy. Median follow-up time was 117 months and most men (>80 %) were diagnosed at age 65 or older. After 10 years of follow-up, 24 % had died of prostate cancer and another 31 % of other causes. The detailed risk analysis confirms again the prognostic value of Gleason score, which had the greatest prognostic power of all parameters, but also serum PSA levels and tumour extension in the primary biopsy as prognostic factors. Importantly, the prognostic value of serum PSA was relatively independent from tumour grade, which constituted the basis of the mortality figures provided by the authors, which include patient age, tumour grade and PSA risk groups. It is a strength of this study that the Gleason score used here is up to contemporary standards, and the addition of serum PSA as an independent prognostic parameter in conservatively treated localised prostate cancer patients has merits. However, the restrictions of follow-up time, the rather elderly patient population and data from other studies that have meanwhile demonstrated the benefits of active treatment for localised prostate cancer somewhat limit the value of these results for modern patient handling.

Bill-Axelson et al. conducted the Scandinavian Prostate Cancer Group Study Number 4 (*SPCGS4*) and compared the outcomes of watchful waiting to radical prostatectomy in patients with early cancer. The patients had to be younger than 75 years and a suspected life expectancy of more than 10 years. Early cancer was defined as a localised tumour (T0D, T1 or T2) with good to moderate differentiation according to the classical WHO definition, a negative bone scan and a serum PSA below 50 ng/ml. In 1999, all cases were subjected to a central review of tumour grade according to the Gleason system. Three-hundred-forty men were randomised to radical prostatectomy and 348 men were assigned to watchful waiting (WW). After a median follow-up time (range 3 weeks to 23 years) of 13.4 years, tumour patient mortality, occurrence of distant metastases and the necessity of palliative treatment were compared. The resultant data was stratified according to patient age and tumour risk groups. The latter were basically defined in analogy to the D'Amico risk groups: *low risk*, Gleason score < 7 (or older WHO grade 1) and serum PSA < 10 ng/ml; *high risk*, serum PSA > 20 ng/ml or Gleason score > 7 and *intermediate*, all in between. The study demonstrated a significantly higher cumulative general death rate at 18 years in the watchful waiting group (68.9 % vs. 56.1 %) with a relative risk for prostatectomy patients of 0.71 ($p < 0.001$). Also, tumour-specific death rates were higher in the WW group at 18 years (28.7 % vs. 17.7 %). Of the 247 deceased patients in the WW group, younger age (<65 years) was associated with tumour-specific death (51 % vs. 30 %). In the group of low-risk tumours, 5.6 % of all WW patients experienced tumour-specific death; in patients with moderate tumour risk, 14.4 % succumbed to their tumour; and the high-risk group displayed 8.3 % tumour-specific death. The authors conclude that radical prostatectomy substantially reduces patient mortality, especially in younger or intermediate-risk patients; however, they also acknowledge that a large proportion of long-term survivors in the WW arm of their study have not required palliative treatment [12]. This extensive study provides a wealth of data for the current discussion on deferred or local therapies, even though the cohort size precludes in-depth analyses of patient subgroups. However, the definition of risk groups is not stringent, since the low-risk group uses an alloy of Gleason score (from 1999) and Mostofi-based WHO grading, and it is unclear how this Gleason grading would translate in contemporary practice which is based upon the ISUP recommendation of 2005 [13]. In this study, the main step of tumour-specific mortality increase according to tumour risk groups is from the low-risk to the moderate-risk group, suggesting that the latter would profit more from active therapy. As the authors discuss, the important finding of patients with a considerable tumour load that still belong to the group of long-term survivors without curative therapy underscores the importance to generate better prognostic tools to identify these patients prospectively. Apparently, the risk groups used in this study have a certain discriminative power but do not suffice.

An apparently very similar trial to compare the outcomes of radical prostatectomy vs. watchful waiting was the Prostate Cancer Intervention Versus Observation

Trial (*PIVOT*) [14]. The inclusion criteria were nearly identical (localised cancer, PSA < 50 ng/ml, life expectancy >10 years, negative bone scan) but had no restrictions according to tumour grade. Again, a central review of tumour grade was conducted and additionally PSA testing was centralised. Primary and secondary outcomes were overall and prostate cancer-specific survival. In total, 731 patients with a mean age of 67 years and a medium serum PSA of 7.8 ng/ml were recruited and randomised to radical prostatectomy (*n* = 364) or watchful waiting (*n* = 367). The median follow-up time of this study was 10.0 years. Comparing both strategies, the authors did not find significant differences in primary or secondary outcome, which needs to be interpreted with extreme caution. First, the follow-up time may be too short to come to significant conclusions. Second, there is treatment contamination in the nontreatment arm. Maybe most important, the relatively high prevalence of serious diseases that produced Charlson comorbidity scores of 1 or greater in almost half the men may significantly bias the data. Notwithstanding these methodological issues, this study contributes valuable data on WW patients. Overall, 49.9 % of these had died by the end of the study. Death from prostate cancer was assigned in 2.7 % of low-risk patients, 10.8 % of intermediate-risk patients and 17.5 % of high-risk patients, according to D'Amico risk scores [15]. Stratified for Gleason scores alone, patients whose tumours had Gleason scores <7 died in 5.7 % (15/261) of cases, whereas higher Gleason scores conferred an increased mortality of 17.4 % (15/85). Again, in this study, a high rate of patients with high risk tumours have survived even without treatment, but the relatively short follow-up time somewhat hampers this finding. The earlier study of Johansson et al., who had also analysed the long-term follow-up of localised prostate cancer, recognised a markedly increased mortality in patients who had survived the first 15 years, which also suggests that longer follow-up in the PIVOT trial is advisable [16].

Another study that is not exactly in the focus of this overview but ought to be mentioned is the European Randomized Study of Screening for Prostate Cancer (ERSPC) [17, 18]. This trial aimed to clarify the effects of screening on the course of clinical prostate cancer. This multinational study provided the first proof that PSA screening reduces mortality of prostate cancer. The current update (conference communication, FH Schröder, Lancet 2014 in press) demonstrated a relative risk reduction of 21 %. The number of patients needed to screen (NNS) dropped from 936 to 871 and the number needed to treat (NNT) to 27. This results in an absolute reduction of prostate cancer mortality to 1.28/1,000 men.

Even though all of these studies have idiosyncratic differences regarding patient selection (e.g. PSA screened, non-screened, ethnicity, etc.) and study design and follow-up time, these studies unite in the recognition of prostate cancer as a malignancy that shows on average long courses with considerable individual variations with patient age and tumour grade as leading prognostic parameters. Serum PSA was not systematically analysed in all of these studies but also appears to be a major prognostic factor. These data also indicate that a strictly conservative approach may be considered for some patients, as the existence of non-treated long-term survivors suggests, but this decision has to be made very consciously considering patient age, remaining life expectancy and tumour parameters (grade, extent, serum PSA) to minimise misclassifications. Obviously, patients with higher tumour grade and younger age would benefit the most from active treatment, as they are at higher risk of tumour-associated death. Conversely, older patients with pre-existing morbidity and low-grade tumours may possibly not experience the oncologic benefit of active therapy, which may necessitate a life span of over 15 years, as the data from Albertsen suggests. For the extremes, the decision upon the most appropriate treatment strategy may be relatively easy; however, for the group of medium-aged patients with low- to intermediate-risk tumours, this is quite unclear. To answer this question, further prospective trials are needed. One of these, in which the author is actively involved as the coordinator of the reference pathology, is the PREFERE trial [19, 20]. This aims to compare the outcomes of patients with low to early-intermediate-risk tumours, which are randomised either to radical prostatectomy, external beam radiation, brachytherapy or active surveillance. Active surveillance is the deliberate attempt to postpone a potentially curative therapy to the latest possible time point and thus should be not be confused with the passive concept of watchful waiting. The therapeutic concept to postpone therapy has gradually evolved based on the long-term observational data on prostate cancer and aims to prevent overtreatment and to spare the patient the burden of treatment-associated morbidity as long as possible [21–23]. However, this strategy may be restricted to patients with low-grade tumours only and requires a well-educated and – possibly most important – compliant patient that obeys the follow-up regimen including repetitive re-biopsies. Therefore the use of active surveillance may best be placed in strictly controlled studies. The PREFERE trial plans to observe the patients over 13 years following inclusion and will not only compare patient mortality but also the quality of life, which is of increasing interest with growing patient awareness. A greater enthusiasm of practising urologists to support this study would be desirable to successfully complete this important prospective study.

1.5 The Concepts of Clinically Different Prostate Cancer Variants

Many authors differentiate between insignificant, indolent, latent and lethal prostate cancer, terms that are not always used correctly. The obviously diverse clinical faces of prostate and the difficulties to predict the individual course have early prompted attempts to define a definitely harmless variant of cancer that does not interfere with the patient's normal life span. Stamey was among the first to define this group as "insignificant prostate cancer" [24]. His definition stemming from an analysis of incidental prostate cancer findings in cystoprostatectomy specimens included tumour grade (Gleason score 6) and a tumour volume below 0.5 cc. The widely used criteria for insignificant cancer from Epstein et al. also include an organ-confined tumour (pT2) with a tumour volume of 0.5 cc and a Gleason score ≤ 6 (no Gleason pattern 4!) [25]. To use this definition with absolute certainty would necessitate a "diagnostic prostatectomy"; hence its translation to needle biopsy-based diagnostics is not without problems, due to inevitable sampling bias. Also, as Lawrence Klotz had pointed out recently, the cut-off of 0.5 cc tumour volume may be too narrow and restrictive [22]. The ERSPC study assumed an overdiagnosis of 50 % in the screening arm in comparison to the clinically detected patient group and suggested a new cut-off value of 1.3 cc to define insignificant tumours [26], which equates to a diameter of 1.4 cm of an ellipsoid tumour, in comparison to 1 cm (0.5 cc). Apparently, there is also some definition overlap of insignificant, indolent and minimal prostate cancer [27]. Van der Kwast had recently re-analysed the issue of demarcation of insignificant and significant prostate cancer and suggests five hypothetical forms of prostate cancer [28]. *Indolent carcinomas* (type I) are supposed to remain in the latent, clinically unapparent phase and constitute the majority of cases found at autopsy, if carefully analysed. *Low-risk tumours* (type II) may stay latent for a longer time but will eventually be detected by PSA screening or digital rectal examination (DRE). Low-risk tumours with grade progression (type III) will escape the zone of latency earlier and become a significant tumour. A fourth group of tumours, de novo high grade (type IV), is supposed to develop as a primary high-grade tumour and will stay latent only for a short while. Finally, a rare set of *early-onset tumours* (type V) arises in young men and will also show a more aggressive course. As tempting as this proposal is, it is not possible to translate this model into clinical practice in every instance, since the groups proposed here overlap significantly. A biopsy-detected tumour with a minute amount of Gleason pattern 4 in a 60-year-old patient may either belong to group I, II or III. As of yet, it is unclear if we can diagnose these tumour categories with certainty in each patient.

1.6   Estimates of Prostate Cancer Aggressiveness: Prognostic Factors in Needle Biopsies

In most cases, the diagnosis of prostate cancer will have been made on needle biopsy following an abnormal DRE or elevated serum PSA levels; therefore, this overview will be restricted to prognostic factors in needle biopsy-detected cases. *Tumour volume* has repetitively been confirmed as a prognostic factor, even if not multivariately significant following radical prostatectomy [29]. Of course, the tumour extent sampled in systematic biopsies does correlate with tumour size seen after surgery [30]. Consequently, the number of positive biopsies and the tumour extent are predictive of adverse pathological parameters following radical prostatectomy and patient outcome [31, 32].

Tumour multifocality is difficult to evaluate on needle biopsies alone, and a close correlation with radiological (MRT) findings may be helpful to clarify this issue, but this is currently not a standard of care. It is long known that prostate cancer is commonly multifocal [33]. Byar et al. reviewed 208 prostatectomy specimens and found 85 % of cases with multifocal tumours [34]. As can be expected, they also found tumour multifocality associated with other parameters of progressive disease, e.g. extraprostatic extension and seminal vesicle infiltration. Rice et al. aimed to clarify the biological potency of unifocal tumours [35]. This is important since these rarer unifocal prostate tumours appear as ideal targets for focal therapy approaches but have not been sufficiently characterised. They confirmed a rate of 8.9 % unifocal tumours in their cohort of 1,056 patients. Surprisingly, this highly powered study showed higher Gleason scores and adverse outcomes for the group of unifocal tumours. First, this illustrates the necessity to re-analyse previous findings in contemporary contexts (PSA screening), but it also shows that unifocal tumours are at least as aggressive as multifocal tumours and should be extensively staged, before the option of focal therapy is considered. It can be speculated that unifocal tumours belong to a larger extent to the de novo high-grade group of prostate cancer.

Tumour grade is the best verified and strongest prognostic parameter in prostate cancer. The pronounced morphological heterogeneity of prostate cancer has been a challenge to pathologists in their attempts to categorise this tumour into biologically meaningful subgroups. Since its first description by Donald Gleason in 1966, the prognostic power of grading prostate cancer primarily by its architectural patterns, taking this marked heterogeneity into account, has repetitively been confirmed and has meanwhile become the global standard [36]. Since it was not developed to be primarily applied to needle biopsies at that time, minor alterations in its use were noticed over time and led the International Society of Urological Pathology (ISUP) in 2005 to convene on this matter to formulate a contemporary update on Gleason grading, which is now regarded as the new standard [13]. The updated Gleason grading according the ISUP has meanwhile been well received among practising pathologist. In a recent poll of the European Network of Uropathology (ENUP), 93 % of participants reported to use this system [37].

Use of the revised Gleason grade has led to certain improvements in prostate diagnostics. Particularly in Germany, where other grading systems had long prevailed, the correct use of Gleason grading was unevenly distributed before the World Health Organisation (WHO) adopted Gleason grading in 2004, and the discussion on the introduction of the revised grading a year later has helped to promote Gleason grading in Germany. The ISUP grading has helped to harmonise Gleason scores between needle biopsies and radical prostatectomies, at the expense of a Gleason shift towards higher grades [38, 39]. Gleason scores of 5 or lower are not diagnosed anymore in biopsies, even though the ISUP recommendation does not explicitly forbid it. Some voices had criticised the ISUP update, for no urologists were involved in this transformation. Also, it may have a significant impact on patient handling, as all prognostic schemes that were built using the "old" Gleason system may not be correct anymore. This is half true, since we have observed a Gleason shift in some laboratories, whereas others were less affected, if they had practised a more modern interpretation of the traditional Gleason patterns beforehand. In this sense, it is important to realise that the ISUP recommendation was not something totally new that creative spirits had made up at the green table but the consensus of common practice of opinion leaders in the field, clearly with a predominance of northern American pathologists. That this Gleason shift may indeed be very modest can be seen in the data of Zareba et al., who compared Gleason scores of a larger cohort before and after 2005 and found significantly higher scores after the ISUP recommendation, albeit with the minor difference of a mean Gleason score of 6.34

(old) vs. 6.49 (new), which is probably irrelevant and merely underscores that the practice has not changed markedly in this laboratory due to the ISUP publication [40]. Several studies have confirmed the prognostic value of the ISUP grading and particularly the difference between the old and the new definition of Gleason patterns 3 and 4 [39, 41].

Although nuclear morphology is a prognostic factor in many grading systems of human tumours, the Gleason system does not incorporate this. The traditional German variation of the old Mostofi-based WHO grading system ("Helpap grading") combined architectural and cytological criteria in a scoring system to derive a final grade [42]. Although this grading system is competitive and powerful, it has never gained international recognition but is still widely used as an adjunct grading system in Germany. The fact that we do encounter problematic cases in Gleason grading which exhibits a marked discrepancy of a high-grade nuclear morphology and a low-grade growth pattern cannot be disputed. In smaller series it has been shown that the dual use of Gleason and Helpap grading may have added value in the prognostication of patients [43–45]. Possibly, but this is speculative, the relevance of nuclear morphology needs to be recognised in further studies and incorporated in a later update of Gleason grading.

Perineural invasion (Pn1) is seen in virtually every prostatectomy specimen that has been carefully worked up; hence, its prognostic value is limited. This was supposed to be different in needle biopsies, in which the diagnosis of Pn1 was assumed predictive of larger tumours on radical prostatectomy. However, many pathologists do not routinely search for perineural invasion or simply overlook it, e.g. mistake it for collagenous nodules. Harnden et al. undertook a comprehensive meta-analysis of studies on Pn1 in prostate cancer, which concluded that although Pn1 is associated with other poor prognostic indicators and probably hinting towards active therapy, however, its independent prognostic value remains still unclear, necessitating further studies [46].

Intraductal carcinoma is conceptionally a post-invasive lesion that represents invasive carcinoma that happens to spread in pre-existing prostatic ducts. Morphologically, distended ducts, which retain a basal cell layer, are filled with atypical cribriform or solid tumour cell proliferates, often with a central comedo necrosis [47]. This propensity to spread within ducts is apparently restricted to tumours of high Gleason scores, which makes the correct diagnosis of this lesion important. This concept also implicates that the diagnosis of isolated intraductal carcinoma, if made with confidence, is indicative of invasive carcinoma elsewhere. It is, however, not clear if immediate therapy for suspected high-grade invasive tumour or immediate re-biopsy is most appropriate. A small cohort of 21 cases with isolated intraductal cancer in the absence of invasive cancer on biopsy was treated surgically. In the radical prostatectomy specimens, an invasive carcinoma was seen in 90 % of cases and two cases had only the intraductal neoplasm. Of the invasive carcinomas, the median Gleason score was 8, and 37 % of specimens had a primary or secondary Gleason pattern of 5, which underscores that intraductal tumours are usually of higher grade [48]. It is, however, problematic that we do not have a universally accepted morphological definition of intraductal carcinoma [49, 50]. It can be seen that some pathologists assign a Gleason score (mostly 8) even to isolated intraductal carcinomas, which is highly questionable, given the potential failure rate of >10 %. In my opinion, tumour grading should be restricted to invasive tumours.

Molecular prognostic markers do currently not play a role in histopathological diagnosis. In challenging cases, pathologists widely use a panel of *diagnostic markers* to confirm or rule out a diagnosis of cancer; the most commonly used are basal cell markers (e.g. p63, CK5/6) and positive markers of neoplastic change (e.g. AMACR). Apart from this, immunohistochemical prognostic markers are highly dubious, since they usually lack a prospective validation. It is a common misconception that markers that have been found as prognostic indicators in a retrospective analysis can simply be used prospectively, and it holds even true for markers that have repetitively been shown to be prognostic, e.g. the proliferation marker Ki-67. Most problematic is the standardisation of the assays, which is a true challenge for a semiquantitative technique like immunohistochemistry [51].

The same applies for *DNA cytometry*. This is a technique to determine the DNA content of cells that detect aberrations from the physiological state of diploidy. In virtually all tumours, aneuploidy is associated with increased tumour aggressiveness and prostate cancer is no exception here. Still, the suggested use of DNA cytometry to identify active surveillance patients is highly questionable, since it is not based on supporting data of prospective studies but on a wealth of retrospective studies, with the majority stemming from the pre-ISUP 2005 era [52–55]. Clearly, prospective trials are necessary to elucidate the prognostic value of DNA cytometry in localised prostate cancer.

Prognostic transcript signatures are new diagnostic tools, which are commercially available, that make use of the fact that mRNA levels can better be quantified in a multiplexed fashion than protein expression. It cannot be disputed that these tests are a highly interesting option to improve our diagnostics; however, further validation in prospective trials is needed to confirm the clinical value and their applicability [56–58]. Especially, the unavoidable issue of sampling bias and tumour heterogeneity and its influence on the results of these tests need attention. It is not unlikely that these biases may also be strong confounders in molecular testing, as has been shown for renal cancer, where either a favourable or an unfavourable test result could be retrieved from analysing different parts of the very same tumour [59].

1.7 The Reliability of Prostate Biopsy Diagnostics: Can Pathology Be Trusted?

Despite the remarkable developments of radiological techniques, pathologists provide the tissue-based gold standard of diagnostics and remain a core discipline in modern oncology. But what accuracy can be expected from histopathology? What is the value of a second opinion? Recently, it was suggested from the ERSPC data that pathologists would underestimate "the true degree of prostate cancer aggressiveness" in 25–30 % of cases [60]. This statement is unfortunate, as it blames a single discipline for the failure of a diagnostic strategy that clearly rests on two disciplines: one that takes the sample and the other that looks at it. Clearly, what is not sampled in the biopsy cannot be diagnosed by histology. It is beyond this little chapter to discuss the issue of sampling bias and rates of successfully detected carcinomas with varying schemes. In short, the number of detected carcinomas rises with the number of biopsies taken, however, at the expense to increase the detection of insignificant tumours. Therefore, patients should be aware that a single core of Gleason 6 tumour in a classical sextant biopsy has a different biological potential than a comparable finding in an extended saturation scheme [61]. But this is more stochastic than biology. It is a bit of a dilemma in which radiological techniques will hopefully be eventually helpful: the information gained about a tumour will be more precise with an increasing number of biopsies. The most accurate would be the complete analysis of the removed organ, which is of course in stark contrast to the aim to be least invasive.

The *diagnosis of malignancy* itself does not appear to be problematic. The introduction of diagnostic immunohistochemistry has been very helpful here. Still, we can expect that one to two percent of carcinomas will be overlooked, mostly minute foci of low-grade (Gleason score 6) tumours, often of rare types (e.g. pseudohyperplastic, macroacinar, foamy, etc.) [62]. Small foci of atypical glands (ASAP) are equally problematic, even in the hands of experts, which may have kappa values as low as 0.39 in this setting [63]. But since the diagnosis of ASAP will usually be followed by a re-biopsy, this is highly unlikely to harm the patient. However, a second opinion may spare the patient an unnecessary repeat biopsy.

The interobserver variability of Gleason scores has been extensively analysed in numerous studies. These are nicely summarised by Singh et al., who present their own data in the context of other studies (see their Table 5) [64]. Not surprising, experts in genitourinary pathology show a higher degree of concordance than general pathologists [65, 66]. As one can expect from a human-based pattern analysis, there is a considerable interobserver variation, and the kappa values in these studies often revolve around 0.5–0.7, which is quite good. One must bear in mind, that many of these interobserver comparisons analysed a particularly tricky set of lesions and that the rate of correctly classified cases in normal practice is unremarkable. This is also one of the first results of the PREFERE trial that the vast majority of cases (80 %) that underwent the mandatory second opinion can be confirmed and included in the study. Not all cases of study exclusion by reference pathology were due to true mistakes but also due to missing data (e.g. on tumour length) or misinterpretation of the pathology report by clinicians in the study centre. Clearly, pathologists have to understand the necessity to provide a detailed and thorough report on every biopsy received in order to convey as much information as possible. The "old school" approach, which may still rarely be encountered, that once a focus of carcinoma is identified anywhere in the case, the remaining biopsies can be looked at briefly at low power is not sufficient anymore – but the majority of pathologists know this by now.

Conclusions

In summary, even with nowadays' diagnostic tools, it remains difficult to predict the individual clinical course or to really know what will happen if nothing would be done therapeutically. A simple answer does not suffice, and this delegates a lot of responsibility on the shoulders of the counselling clinician and the increasingly knowledgeable patient to consider the interplay of the factors of the patient (as biological age and remaining life expectancy), parameters of biopsy representativity, para-clinical parameters (particularly serum PSA) and, probably most important, tumour biological parameters from the histology report (and possibly adjunct molecular testing in the future) in the prediction of the individual course. Unfortunately, this matter remains a challenge, and a simple answer to the initial question, what would happen if nothing would be done, cannot be given.

References

1. Siegel R, et al. Cancer statistics, 2014. CA Cancer J Clin. 2014;64(1):9–29.
2. Carter HB, et al. Gleason score 6 adenocarcinoma: should it be labeled as cancer? J Clin Oncol. 2012;30(35):4294–6.
3. Gaynor EP. Zur Frage des Prostatakrebses. Virchows Arch. 1938;301(3):602–52.
4. Breslow N, et al. Latent carcinoma of prostate at autopsy in seven areas. The International Agency for Research on Cancer, Lyons, France. Int J Cancer. 1977;20(5):680–8.
5. Sakr WA, et al. High grade prostatic intraepithelial neoplasia (HGPIN) and prostatic adenocarcinoma between the ages of 20–69: an autopsy study of 249 cases. In Vivo. 1994;8(3):439–43.
6. Zlotta AR, et al. Prevalence of prostate cancer on autopsy: cross-sectional study on unscreened Caucasian and Asian men. J Natl Cancer Inst. 2013;105(14):1050–8.
7. Kaufmann E. Lehrbuch der speziellen pathologischen Anatomie, vol. 2. Berlin: Reimer; 1911.
8. Chodak GW, et al. Results of conservative management of clinically localized prostate cancer. N Engl J Med. 1994;330(4):242–8.
9. Albertsen PC, Hanley JA, Fine J. 20-year outcomes following conservative management of clinically localized prostate cancer. JAMA. 2005;293(17):2095–101.
10. Albertsen PC, et al. Competing risk analysis of men aged 55 to 74 years at diagnosis managed conservatively for clinically localized prostate cancer. JAMA. 1998;280(11):975–80.
11. Cuzick J, et al. Long-term outcome among men with conservatively treated localised prostate cancer. Br J Cancer. 2006;95(9):1186–94.
12. Bill-Axelson A, et al. Radical prostatectomy or watchful waiting in early prostate cancer. N Engl J Med. 2014;370(10):932–42.
13. Epstein JI, et al. The 2005 International Society of Urological Pathology (ISUP) Consensus Conference on Gleason Grading of Prostatic Carcinoma. Am J Surg Pathol. 2005;29(9):1228–42.
14. Wilt TJ, et al. Radical prostatectomy versus observation for localized prostate cancer. N Engl J Med. 2012;367(3):203–13.
15. D'Amico AV, et al. Biochemical outcome after radical prostatectomy, external beam radiation therapy, or interstitial radiation therapy for clinically localized prostate cancer. JAMA. 1998;280(11):969–74.
16. Johansson JE, et al. Natural history of early, localized prostate cancer. JAMA. 2004;291(22):2713–9.
17. Schroder FH, et al. Screening and prostate-cancer mortality in a randomized European study. N Engl J Med. 2009;360(13):1320–8.

18. Schroder FH, et al. Prostate-cancer mortality at 11 years of follow-up. N Engl J Med. 2012;366(11):981–90.
19. Kristiansen G, et al. The importance of pathology in the German prostate cancer study PREFERE. Pathologe. 2013;34(5):449–62.
20. Stockle M, Bussar-Maatz R. Localised prostate cancer: the PREFERE trial. Z Evid Fortbild Qual Gesundhwes. 2012;106(5):333–5; discussion 335.
21. Klotz L. Active surveillance not only reduces morbidity, It saves lives. Oncology (Williston Park). 2013;27(6):522, 593.
22. Klotz L, Emberton M. Management of low risk prostate cancer: active surveillance and focal therapy. Curr Opin Urol. 2014;24(3):270–9.
23. Thomsen FB, et al. Active surveillance for clinically localized prostate cancer – a systematic review. J Surg Oncol. 2014;109(8):830–5.
24. Stamey TA, et al. Localized prostate cancer. Relationship of tumor volume to clinical significance for treatment of prostate cancer. Cancer. 1993;71(3 Suppl):933–8.
25. Epstein JI, et al. Pathologic and clinical findings to predict tumor extent of nonpalpable (stage T1c) prostate cancer. JAMA. 1994;271(5):368–74.
26. Wolters T, et al. A critical analysis of the tumor volume threshold for clinically insignificant prostate cancer using a data set of a randomized screening trial. J Urol. 2011;185(1):121–5.
27. Bangma CH, Roobol MJ. Defining and predicting indolent and low risk prostate cancer. Crit Rev Oncol Hematol. 2012;83(2):235–41.
28. Van der Kwast TH, Roobol MJ. Defining the threshold for significant versus insignificant prostate cancer. Nat Rev Urol. 2013;10(8):473–82.
29. Wolters T, et al. Should pathologists routinely report prostate tumour volume? The prognostic value of tumour volume in prostate cancer. Eur Urol. 2010;57(5):821–9.
30. Zavaski ME, et al. Prostate biopsy volume predicts final tumor volume. Conn Med. 2014;78(3):167–72.
31. Sebo TJ, et al. The percent of cores positive for cancer in prostate needle biopsy specimens is strongly predictive of tumor stage and volume at radical prostatectomy. J Urol. 2000;163(1):174–8.
32. Freedland SJ, et al. Percent prostate needle biopsy tissue with cancer is more predictive of biochemical failure or adverse pathology after radical prostatectomy than prostate specific antigen or Gleason score. J Urol. 2002;167(2 Pt 1):516–20.
33. Gaynor EP. Zur Frages des Prostatakrebses. Virchows Archiv. 1938;301(3): 602–52.
34. Byar DP, Mostofi FK. Carcinoma of the prostate: prognostic evaluation of certain pathologic features in 208 radical prostatectomies. Examined by the step-section technique. Cancer. 1972;30(1):5–13.
35. Rice KR, et al. Clinicopathological behavior of single focus prostate adenocarcinoma. J Urol. 2009;182(6):2689–94.
36. Gleason DF. Classification of prostatic carcinomas. Cancer Chemother Rep. 1966;50(3):125–8.
37. Egevad L, et al. Standardization of Gleason grading among 337 European pathologists. Histopathology. 2013;62(2):247–56.
38. Helpap B, Egevad L. The significance of modified Gleason grading of prostatic carcinoma in biopsy and radical prostatectomy specimens. Virchows Arch. 2006;449(6):622–7.
39. Uemura H, et al. Usefulness of the 2005 International Society of Urologic Pathology Gleason grading system in prostate biopsy and radical prostatectomy specimens. BJU Int. 2009;103(9):1190–4.
40. Zareba P, et al. The impact of the 2005 International Society of Urological Pathology (ISUP) consensus on Gleason grading in contemporary practice. Histopathology. 2009;55(4):384–91.
41. Dong F, et al. Impact on the clinical outcome of prostate cancer by the 2005 international society of urological pathology modified Gleason grading system. Am J Surg Pathol. 2012;36(6):838–43.
42. Helpap B, et al. Classification, histologic and cytologic grading and regression grading of prostate cancer. Urologe A. 1985;24(3):156–9.

43. Helpap B, Kollermann J. Combined histoarchitectural and cytological biopsy grading improves grading accuracy in low-grade prostate cancer. Int J Urol. 2012;19(2):126–33.
44. Helpap B, et al. Improving the reproducibility of the Gleason scores in small foci of prostate cancer–suggestion of diagnostic criteria for glandular fusion. Pathol Oncol Res. 2012;18(3):615–21.
45. Helpap B, et al. Significance of Gleason grading of low-grade carcinoma of the prostate with therapeutic option of active surveillance. Urol Int. 2013;90(1):17–23.
46. Harnden P, et al. The prognostic significance of perineural invasion in prostatic cancer biopsies: a systematic review. Cancer. 2007;109(1):13–24.
47. Robinson B, Magi-Galluzzi C, Zhou M. Intraductal carcinoma of the prostate. Arch Pathol Lab Med. 2012;136(4):418–25.
48. Robinson BD, Epstein JI. Intraductal carcinoma of the prostate without invasive carcinoma on needle biopsy: emphasis on radical prostatectomy findings. J Urol. 2010;184(4):1328–33.
49. Guo CC, Epstein JI. Intraductal carcinoma of the prostate on needle biopsy: Histologic features and clinical significance. Mod Pathol. 2006;19(12):1528–35.
50. Cohen RJ, et al. A proposal on the identification, histologic reporting, and implications of intraductal prostatic carcinoma. Arch Pathol Lab Med. 2007;131(7):1103–9.
51. Kristiansen G. Diagnostic and prognostic molecular biomarkers for prostate cancer. Histopathology. 2012;60(1):125–41.
52. Bocking A, et al. Algorithm for a DNA-cytophotometric diagnosis and grading of malignancy. Anal Quant Cytol. 1984;6(1):1–8.
53. Bocking A, et al. Cytology of prostatic carcinoma. Quantification and validation of diagnostic criteria. Anal Quant Cytol. 1984;6(2):74–88.
54. Schroder F, et al. Clinical utility of cellular DNA measurements in prostate carcinoma. Consensus Conference on Diagnosis and Prognostic Parameters in Localized Prostate Cancer. Stockholm, Sweden, May 12-13, 1993. Scand J Urol Nephrol Suppl. 1994;162:51–63; discussion 15–27.
55. Wang N, et al. Evaluation of tumor heterogeneity of prostate carcinoma by flow- and image DNA cytometry and histopathological grading. Anal Cell Pathol. 2000;20(1):49–62.
56. Cuzick J. Prognostic value of a cell cycle progression score for men with prostate cancer. Recent Results Cancer Res. 2014;202:133–40.
57. Knezevic D, et al. Analytical validation of the Oncotype DX prostate cancer assay – a clinical RT-PCR assay optimized for prostate needle biopsies. BMC Genomics. 2013;14:690.
58. Wu CL, et al. Development and validation of a 32-gene prognostic index for prostate cancer progression. Proc Natl Acad Sci U S A. 2013;110(15):6121–6.
59. Gerlinger M, et al. Intratumor heterogeneity and branched evolution revealed by multiregion sequencing. N Engl J Med. 2012;366(10):883–92.
60. Schroder FH. Screening for prostate cancer: current status of ERSPC and screening-related issues. Recent Results Cancer Res. 2014;202:47–51.
61. Villa L, et al. The number of cores taken in patients diagnosed with a single microfocus at initial biopsy is a major predictor of insignificant prostate cancer. J Urol. 2013;189(3):854–9.
62. Wolters T, et al. False-negative prostate needle biopsies: frequency, histopathologic features, and follow-up. Am J Surg Pathol. 2010;34(1):35–43.
63. Van der Kwast TH, et al. Variability in diagnostic opinion among pathologists for single small atypical foci in prostate biopsies. Am J Surg Pathol. 2010;34(2):169–77.
64. Singh RV, et al. Interobserver reproducibility of Gleason grading of prostatic adenocarcinoma among general pathologists. Indian J Cancer. 2011;48(4):488–95.
65. Allsbrook Jr WC, et al. Interobserver reproducibility of Gleason grading of prostatic carcinoma: urologic pathologists. Hum Pathol. 2001;32(1):74–80.
66. Allsbrook Jr WC, et al. Interobserver reproducibility of Gleason grading of prostatic carcinoma: general pathologist. Hum Pathol. 2001;32(1):81–8.

Is Focal Prostate Therapy Just Psychotherapy? Surveillance Versus Focal Therapy: Pros and Cons

2

Shiro Saito

Contents

Prostate cancer is usually a slow-growing cancer and mostly found in relatively old men. Does it need to be treated completely, can it be treated incompletely with maintaining good quality of life (QOL), or even can it remain untreated? To answer this question is not easy because the progression of the disease is difficult to estimate and the patient's life expectancy is unknown. But progression of prostate cancer can be roughly estimated with initial cancer character, such as initial prostate-specific antigen (PSA) level, Gleason score, clinical stage, or positive biopsy core rate. The patient's life expectancy can be estimated from his age and existence of complications. When the prostate cancer seems to have an aggressive feature, or it rises in younger men, the disease may develop some unfavorable events in the future. That kind of cancer must be treated completely at the time of diagnosis. Most of the other patients have disease that won't disturb their QOL or shorten their life and can be kept untreated and surveyed. What will you do for patients whose disease is difficult to guess whether it will commit wicked deed in the future

S. Saito, MD
Department of Urology, National Hospital Organization Tokyo Medical Center,
2-5-1 Higashigaoka Meguro-ku, Tokyo 152-8902, Japan
e-mail: saitoshr@netjoy.ne.jp

© Springer International Publishing Switzerland 2015   19
S. Thüroff, C.G. Chaussy (eds.), *Focal Therapy of Prostate Cancer:*
An Emerging Strategy for Minimally Invasive, Staged Treatment,
DOI 10.1007/978-3-319-14160-2_2

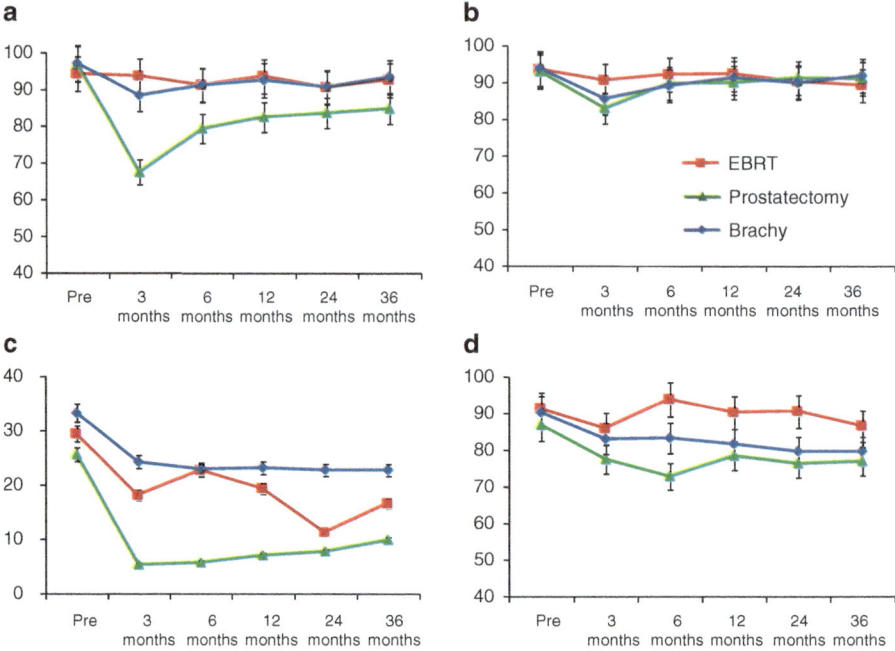

Fig. 2.1 EPIC QOL analysis of urinary function (**a**), urinary bother (**b**), sexual function (**c**), and sexual bother (**d**) for prostate cancer patient who underwent external beam radiotherapy (■), radical prostatectomy (▲), and permanent brachytherapy (◆)

or not? Those cases may be good candidates for focal treatment. With focal therapy, QOL is acceptably maintained, and the life may not be shortened with the disease.

Does focal therapy for localized prostate cancer work just psychologically? Maybe no, but the answer is unknown. Focal therapy may relate to good tumor control. But there are no randomized studies that compare disease-specific survival of surveillance and focal therapy.

Do patients with surveillance have no adverse events? Not always. They sometimes have anxiety that they have cancer in their body and that it is not treated. Are patients who have urinary incontinence or erectile dysfunction related to radical prostatectomy always unhappy? Not always. Even with treatment-related adverse events, patients are not always having a hard time with the symptoms and not always having grudge against the treatment that they have undergone. According to the research for health-related QOL after prostate cancer treatment with Expanded Prostate Cancer Index Composite (EPIC) questionnaire [1], patients who underwent radical prostatectomy have low urinary function score and low sexual function score because of their urinary incontinence and erectile dysfunction. However, the scores for urinary bother and sexual bother gradually recover to previous level even though those functions are still low (Fig. 2.1). From the results of the same questionnaire, even the patients with lifelong adverse events showed their intention of satisfaction to the treatment. It is hard to tell what can make a man happy with the feeling of satisfaction.

Who are the candidates for surveillance or focal therapy? How to follow the patients under the policy of surveillance and how to treat prostate cancer focally? What kinds of satisfaction can patients obtain from surveillance or from focal therapy? Whose QOL is better, patients with surveillance or patients treated with focal therapy? What costs more? Who can live longer? There are a lot of points of pros and cons when discussing about focal therapy for localized prostate cancer.

2.1 What Is Surveillance for Prostate Cancer and How to Perform That?

Prostate cancer surveillance has two different policies that can be defined as active surveillance and non-active surveillance (watchful waiting). Watchful waiting has meant no active treatment until a patient develops evidence of symptomatic disease progression. The goal of this non-interventional approach is to limit morbidity from the disease and therapy. Watchful waiting can be performed to patients with age over 75 or with life expectancy less than 15 years, any clinical stage, any PSA, but Gleason score may be less than 8. They usually won't check PSA, they do not have repeated biopsies, and they will just have palliative treatments when they have symptoms according to progression of the disease [2, 3]. No blood drawing, no biopsy, and no hospital visit may relate to perfect QOL of the patients; however, patients are somewhat exposed to the incidence of prostate cancer death.

Active surveillance with selective delayed definitive therapy attempts to distinguish clinically insignificant cancers from life-threatening cancers while they are still localized to the prostate. With active surveillance, people attempt to avoid over-treatment in the majority of the patients but also to administer curative therapy to selected cases. Active surveillance attempts to perform to patients with ages between 50 and 80, clinically organ-confined disease, PSA less than 15 ng/ml, and Gleason score less than 8. They will check their PSA frequently, they will have repeated biopsy when their PSA rises, and they will have radical treatment when their disease is found as higher grade or more extensive by biopsies [2, 3].

2.2 What Is Focal Therapy for Prostate Cancer and How to Perform That?

Prostate focal therapy is to treat only the cancer site in the prostate. This new policy for treating prostate cancer is a potential bridge between active surveillance and the more aggressive treatment modalities. This treatment has been defined as the "complete ablation for all clinically significant foci within the prostate using a minimally invasive technique with preservation of the sphincter, normal grand tissue and the neurovascular bundles" [4]. The sources of energy to treat cancer focally can be cryotherapy [5, 6], high-intensity focused ultrasound (HIFU) [6], both high-dose-rate (HDR) brachytherapy [7] and low-dose-rate (LDR) brachytherapy [8], radiotherapy, and thermotherapy [9].

What is most important to perform focal therapy is to diagnose the character of cancer accurately and to recognize the exact position of the cancer site. Tumor position can be detected with mapping biopsy [5] and image diagnosis by multiparametric MRI or MRS [10, 11]. According to histological findings of prostatectomy specimens, 67–87 % of prostate has incidence of multifocal disease [12]; however, 80 % of those synchronous secondary tumors occupied less than 0.5 cc volume [13]. Focal therapy cannot eliminate all those multifocal sites, but the destruction of the dominant tumor foci may be adequate to alter the clinical course of prostate cancer; the smaller-volume, low-grade satellite tumors that go undetected and have no impact on the clinical course of prostate cancer remain, just like autopsy cancer [14].

Focal therapy is often performed for local recurrent cases after initial radiation therapy. As the conception for these cases is totally different from initial focal therapy, it won't be discussed here.

2.3   Who Are the Candidates for Surveillance or Focal Therapy?

Criteria for both surveillance and focal therapy are similar. Low-risk prostate cancer, which means cancer with low potential to become advanced disease, can be considered as candidate of surveillance or focal therapy. Low initial PSA (<10 ng/ml), low Gleason score (<7), low clinical stage (<T2c), and small cancer volume are the factors for low-risk cancer. Table 2.1 shows criteria for active surveillance and focal therapy [14, 15]. Clinical stage T1or T2a, PSA <10 ng/ml, Gleason score <7, PSA density <0.15 ng/ml, positive biopsy core rate <33 %, and percent cancer involvement in biopsy core <20–50 % are the criteria mostly used. Additionally, patient age, life expectancy, complications, and family history for prostate cancer can be considered as factors to decide whether to perform surveillance or focal therapy.

If the criteria for surveillance and focal therapy are similar, who are the good candidates for active surveillance and who are going to receive focal therapy? As there is no randomized study comparing these two new policies, there is no correct answer based on the evidence. At this point, the correct answer is a decision of each patient.

2.4   What Is the Advantage or Disadvantage of Surveillance?

The highest advantage of surveillance is that the patients are not treated immediately, and some of them will not need to be treated during their life. With watchful waiting policy, patients do not receive any treatment for cancer. With active surveillance policy, more than half of the patients live without any cancer treatments. These people won't have distress from treatments themselves or adverse events caused by

Table 2.1 Criteria of patient selection for active surveillance and focal therapy in prostate cancer

Active surveillance [15]						Focal therapy [14]
	Johns Hopkins University	University of Toronto	PRIAS	UCSF	Japanese multicenter	Int. Task Force on PCa[a]
cT stage	T1c	T1c	T1c or T2	T1 or T2a	T1c	T1 or T2a
PSA(ng/ml) at diagnosis	ND	≤10–15 (1995–1999) ≤10 (2000–2003)	≤10	≤10	≤20	<10
Gleason score	≤3 + 3	≤3 + 3 (≤3 + 4 in men >70 years until 1999)	≤3 + 3	≤3 + 3	≤3 + 3	No 4 or 5
PSA density (ng/ml/ml)	≤0.15	ND	≤0.2	ND	ND	<0.15
Maximal number of posit cores	2	2 (total core #: any)	2 (8–12 cores)	<33 % biopsy cores	2 (6–12 cores)	<33 % biopsy cores
% cancer involvement	<50 % cancer in any core	<50 % cancer in any core	ND	<50 % cancer in any core	<50 % cancer in any core	<20 % cancer in any core

Abbreviation: *PRIAS* the Prostate Cancer Research International, *UCSF* University of California, San Francisco, *ND* not defined

[a]International Task Force on Prostate Cancer the focal lesion paradigm: proposed clinical biopsy and imaging criteria for focal therapy patient selection. These criteria involve image factor such as single lesion with a maximum size (12 mm), maximum length of capsular contact (10 mm), and no evidence of extraprostatic extension or seminal vesicle invasion

the treatments. QOL will drop down after any kind of prostate cancer treatments, such as radical prostatectomy, external beam radiation therapy, brachytherapy, or androgen ablation therapy. If the patients do not receive any of these treatments, their QOL will not worsen by the treatments. But on the other hand, when watchful waiting patients live long until the cancer progresses and causes hard symptoms, patients may have distress from that and may die from cancer. Randomized comparison of watchful waiting and radical prostatectomy revealed higher cumulative incidence of death from prostate cancer in watchful waiting group [16].

With active surveillance policy, patients may be able to avoid performing curative treatments or may delay the treatments. But they need frequent PSA test and multiple chances of biopsy, and they always need to worry about their disease progression. Moreover, Choo et al. [17] reported that 19 % in 2 years and 33 % in 4 years had disease progression, and Patel et al. [18] reported that 33 % in 5 years and 45 % in 10 years had disease progression, and those patients are recommended to have curative treatment anyhow. As reported by Patel et al. [18], when active surveillance patients did not undergo proper treatment for cancer at the diagnosis of progression, the probability that they remain progressive is statistically higher than those without diagnosis of progression. Active surveillance may be a feasible alternative to initial curative treatment in select patients with favorable, localized prostate cancer. About half of the patients remain free of progression at 10 years, and definitive treatment appeared effective in those with progression [18]. It is important to perceive the disease progression before it turns to incurable disease.

2.5   What Is the Advantage or Disadvantage of Focal Therapy?

Focal therapy for prostate cancer is thought as a potential bridge between active surveillance and the more aggressive treatment modalities such as radical prostatectomy, radiation therapy, etc. What is expected for focal therapy is that it may cure the disease without seeing any adverse events exerting some bad influence to QOL. Thus, the advantage for this treatment is that the patient can obtain good oncologic outcome and also favorable functional outcome. But on the other hand, focal therapy may not treat cancer completely or may continue to some kinds of treatment-related adverse events. Thus, the disadvantage of this treatment is that there is a possibility to be depressed after the treatment with unsuccessful cancer control and with patient's functional damage.

As focal therapy is relatively a new policy for the treatment of prostate cancer, there are no data with long follow-up period. But with short-term data with limited number of cases, focal therapy treated with either cryotherapy [5, 6], HIFU [6], HDR brachytherapy [7], or LDR brachytherapy [8] revealed favorable outcomes, both oncologic and functional. With adequate diagnosis of cancer focus, focal therapy with any of these devices may be able to control cancer locally. And with limited treatment area, focal therapy may not have relevance to any adverse events in urinary, rectal, or sexual function.

Conclusions

Active surveillance and focal therapy are both passive treatment options for localized low-risk prostate cancer. Criteria for both policies are similar, and there is no randomized study to compare these two to create clinical evidence. As PSA is a divine revelation for prostate cancer patients, maintaining PSA at low level with treatment is a good tranquilizer for them. Focal therapy may create low PSA with low incidence of adverse events. Then, performing focal therapy is just for obtaining psychological satisfaction. Randomized study may clarify this answer; however, eliminating the main focus of cancer may provide certain benefit for disease-specific survival compared with surveillance. With surveillance, there is a possibility to miss the point of limit to start treatment not to die from cancer. But still there are many pros and cons.

References

1. Kakehi Y, Takegami Y, Suzukamo Y, et al. Health related quality of life in Japanese men with localized prostate cancer treated with current multiple modalities assessed by a newly developed Japanese version of the expanded prostate cancer index composite. J Urol. 2007;177(5):1856–61.
2. Eastham JA, Scardino PT. Expectant management of prostate cancer. In: Wein AJ, editor. Cambel-Walsh urology. 9th ed. Philadelphia: Saunders; 2007. p. 2947–55.
3. Parker C. Active surveillance of early prostate cancer: rationale, initial results and future developments. Prostate Cancer Prostatic Dis. 2004;7(3):184–7.
4. Crawford ED, Barqawi AB. Targeted focal therapy: a minimally invasive ablation technique for early prostate cancer. Oncology. 2007;21(1):27–32.
5. Sullivan KF, Crawford ED. Target focal therapy for prostate cancer: a review of the literature. Ther Adv Urol. 2009;1(3):149–59.
6. Iberti CT, Mohamed N, Palese MA. A review of focal therapy techniques in prostate cancer: clinical results for high-intensity focused ultrasound and focal cryoablation. Rev Urol. 2011;13(4):196–202.
7. Kamrava M, Chung MP, Kayode O, et al. Focal high-dose-rate brachytherapy: a dosimetric comparison of hemigland vs. conventional whole-gland treatment. Brachytherapy. 2013;12(5):434–41.
8. Cosset JM, Cathelineau X, Wakil G, et al. Focal brachytherapy for selected low-risk prostate cancers: a pilot study. Brachytherapy. 2013;12(4):331–7.
9. Barqawi AB, Krughoff KJ, Eid K. Current challenges in prostate cancer management and the rationale behind targeted focal therapy. Adv Urol. 2012. doi:10.1155/2012/862639.
10. Lee DH, Koo KC, Lee SH, et al. Low-risk prostate cancer patients without visible tumor (T1c) on multi-parametric MRI could qualify for active surveillance candidate even if they did not meet inclusion criteria of active surveillance protocol. Jpn J Clin Oncol. 2013;43(5):553–8.
11. Sartor AO, Hricak H, Wheeler TM, et al. Evaluating localized prostate cancer and identifying candidates for focal therapy. Urology. 2008;72(6 suppl):12–24.
12. Meiers I, Waters D, Bostwick D. Preoperative prediction of multifocal prostate cancer and application of focal therapy: review 2007. Urology. 2007;70(6 suppl):3–8.
13. Wise A, Stamey T, McNeal J, et al. Morphologic and clinical significance of multifocal prostate cancer in radical prostatectomy specimens. Urology. 2002;60(2):264–9.
14. Ward JF, Pisters LL. Considerations for patient selection for focal therapy. Ther Adv Urol. 2013;5(6):330–7.
15. Kakehi Y. Active surveillance as a practical strategy to differentiate lethal and non-lethal prostate cancer subtypes. Asian J Androl. 2012;14(3):361–4.
16. Bill-Axelson A, Holmberg L, Ruutu M. Radical prostatectomy versus watchful waiting in early prostate cancer. N Engl J Med. 2005;352(19):1977–84.
17. Choo R, Klotz L, Danjoux C. Feasible study: watchful waiting for localized low to intermediate grade prostate carcinoma with selective delayed intervention based on prostate specific antigen, histological and/or clinical progression. J Urol. 2002;167(4):1664–9.
18. Patel MI, DeConcini DT, Lopez-Corona E, et al. An analysis of men with clinically localized prostate cancer who deferred definitive therapy. J Urol. 2004;171(4):1520–4.

Definitive Focal Therapy for Prostate Cancer Therapy: What's It and Why Should(nt) We Offer It?

3

Osamu Ukimura, John C. Rewcastle, and Inderbir S. Gill

Contents

3.1 Evolving Concept of Focal Therapy

In contemporary clinical practice, the majority of the solid organ cancers undergo excision or targeted ablation to definitively treat one or more lesions while adjacent healthy tissues are preserved as best as possible. However, until recently, only a few urologists and radiologists have questioned the status quo of definitive local therapy for prostate cancer being a radical whole-gland approach. Patients are often more aggressive in challenging this paradigm. The newly diagnosed prostate cancer patient faces a dilemma of when and how to treat their disease. Many have likely questioned why their doctor does not offer the attractive option of targeted focal therapy of the known cancer with minimizing the treatment-related side effects.

Ward et al. [1] stated that "In as much as focal therapy must not be an excuse to treat men who do not require treatment, our current inability to accurately stage

O. Ukimura (✉) • J.C. Rewcastle • I.S. Gill
USC Institute of Urology, Keck School of Medicine,
University of Southern California, Los Angeles, CA, USA
e-mail: drukimurao@gmail.com; gillindy@gmail.com

© Springer International Publishing Switzerland 2015
S. Thüroff, C.G. Chaussy (eds.), *Focal Therapy of Prostate Cancer:*
An Emerging Strategy for Minimally Invasive, Staged Treatment,
DOI 10.1007/978-3-319-14160-2_3

27

prostate cancer intraprostatically must not be justification to marginalize or dismiss the approach."

We believe that it is the time to make targeted focal therapy a real and responsible treatment option for prostate cancer. This belief is based on the various technologies to a focal therapy approach having evolved and advanced. These technologies are both diagnostic (molecular markers, imaging modalities, biopsy strategies) and therapeutic (ablative technologies such as HIFU and cryoablation). However, their evolutions have largely been independent of one another. A robust program would incorporate these technologies into one comprehensive platform or protocol.

It is hypothesized that focal therapy of prostate cancer could have a beneficial role to cure or control the known cancer without compromising life expectancy while preserving prostate tissue and adjacent tissues, such as the neurovascular bundle or urinary sphincter, thereby minimizing lifetime treatment-related morbidity [2, 3].

All definitive local therapies for prostate cancer are associated with a distinct pattern of change in quality-of-life (QOL) domains related to urinary, sexual, bowel, and hormonal functions [4]. These changes of QOL impact not only patients but also their families, most significantly their spouses or partners.

Active surveillance (AS) has become the standard option for low-grade low-volume cancer [5–7]. Focal therapy has been suggested as an option to avoid the negative impact on QOL by the current standard whole-gland treatment. However, focal therapy is not attractive to all men and has the potential of missing significant disease. It is worthy to debate the difference of the selection criteria for AS and focal therapy strategies. Certainly there will be an overlap with the treatment decision made by the patient in concert with his family and physicians.

Patients with intermediate and perhaps even high-risk disease may also prove to be candidates for focal therapy. If prostate cancer can be accurately diagnosed in terms of Gleason and stage, it may be possible to include such patients as well.

3.2   Who May Have Benefit by Focal Therapy?

There are, in fact, many groups of patients who may benefit from focal therapy.

The incidentally diagnosed low-grade, low-volume localized cancer may not require immediate radical treatment, being suitable for AS. However, if focal therapy could treat the known disease, curing or acceptably controlling the cancer, it would be an appealing option for men who otherwise would be suitable candidates for active surveillance but hold reservations of selecting no therapy against their cancer.

Focal therapy may also benefit men who are already being surveyed actively by longitudinal observation who have repeat biopsy demonstrating progression in either volume or grade to a clinically significant cancer. Focal therapy of the specific location of the biopsy-proven progressed cancer is an appealing less invasive option which may avoid the adverse effects induced by conventional whole-gland radical therapy.

Primary focal therapy may also be effective for initially diagnosed intermediate risk which can be limited in the specific location in the prostate as long as it is clinically identified as an index lesion.

Prostate cancer is usually multifocal. However, the natural history of the multifocal diseases needs to be considered. We believe that the management of multifocal prostate cancers must be multidisciplinary and longitudinal over the lifetime of the patient. An important fact is that even though the patient on AS often has multifocal disease without clinical identification of multifocal disease at the start of AS, the AS strategy often works at least for several years to successfully delay radical treatment. This indirectly supports the potential ability of focal therapy in the patient who has multifocal disease. Importantly, for multifocal prostate cancer, there is an "index lesion," defined as the largest in volume or highest grade in the prostate which dominates the natural history of that patient's prostate cancer [8–10]. If the index lesion was successfully controlled by focal therapy, the other possibly existing multifocal non-index lesions would be unlikely to compromise life expectancy. AS of these remained non-index cancers is applicable after the successful focal therapy of the index cancer. We could hypothesize that such combined protocol of focal therapy with following AS would be a way of longitudinal minimally invasive management strategy of low-intermediate risk prostate cancer.

Few people have discussed the possible role of focal therapy in men with high-risk disease. The risk of locally advanced disease and/or lymph node involvement is not negligible in the man with non-low-risk prostate. However, focal therapy in conjunction with robotic-assisted laparoscopic pelvic lymphadenectomy (for precise staging and additional therapeutic benefit) might be considerable. This may be an attractive option for select men with newly diagnosed high-risk cancer who have significant comorbidities or are very elderly and who may not be candidates for radical invasive therapy. The role of focal therapy in this setting is worthy of debate.

Furthermore, in salvage setting, focal therapy could be beneficial for men who had locally recurred cancer lesion after whole-gland radical therapy. Since the rest of the tissue has already been treated, focal therapy specifically targeting the recurrence offers an appealing option for men who want to minimize the further change from the existing QOL [11, 12].

Immune reactivity induced and enhanced by focal ablation of the local lesions is a unique and promising concept [13–15]. This may support further expanded indications for focal therapy. The local destruction of the cancer cells results in the release of cell materials which were unlikely exposed before the destruction of the cells. Such antigen specific to cancer cells potentially induces the autologous immune system to be effective for not only local control but also systematic immune response to target the circulating cells or metastatic cancer cells. The future role of focal therapy may not be limited to only controlling local disease but may also involve directly or indirectly systematic therapeutics.

3.3   What Is Essential for Successful Focal Therapy?

Improved quality of imaging to visualize suspicious lesions is vital to better characterize the cancer. Modern imaging, such as multiparametric MRI (mp-MRI) and mp-TRUS, could improve the process of prostate cancer localization and staging. Since the focal therapy is image-guided surgery, imaging technique is in fact an essential part of the surgical technique [16, 17].

The primary challenge for focal therapy is intraprostatic staging. Specifically, precise three-dimensional (3D) mapping of the cancer lesions in combination with histologic characterization is essential as are information from biomarkers – most importantly (today) PSA. There has been significant debate about the optimum biopsy strategy before focal therapy. Current standard prostate biopsy practices have significant sampling errors and often do not map all existing cancer.

In order to maximize detection and mapping of clinically significant cancers, contemporary researchers have discussed transperineal template mapping techniques as well as image-targeted biopsy [18, 19]. Imaging potentially improves the process of cancer detection through the ability to visualize and characterize lesions. A higher positive rate for clinically significant cancer of image-targeted biopsy-proven cancers in suspicious areas has been reported using evolving imaging modalities such as advanced TRUS technologies or multiparametric MRI. A recent systematic review of image-targeted biopsy using MRI reported that positive rate of cancer was 30 % (375 of 1,252) in targeted cores versus 7 % (368 of 5,441) in systematic cores. The efficacy (number of clinically significant cancers/number of men biopsied) of targeted biopsy from MRI abnormalities outperformed to that of systematic sampling (70 % vs. 40 %) [20].

Since image guidance facilitates needle delivery to these sites, often missed by routine sextant biopsies and image-visible targets, imaging should be considered a key modality in maximizing the detection of clinically significant cancer as well as minimizing the number of cores taken [21]. However, the estimation of the index cancer volume and prediction of contouring of the index lesion are still challenging, since imaging often underestimates cancer volume [24–26]. As such, in order to achieve complete destruction of the image-visible index lesion, consideration of image-based underestimation needs to be accounted in the planning for ideal therapeutic area of focal therapy. Furthermore, although macroscopic extraprostatic disease may be visualized by modern imaging [25, 26], there is still a challenge in staging of microscopic extraprostatic disease [22]. Since significant percentage of candidate for surgery has finally revealed extraprostatic disease, there is definitive limitation for precise staging of microscopic extraprostatic extension in contemporary practice. Clearly, improved nomogram to precisely predict the microscopic extraprostatic disease is awaited using modern imaging.

There are critical preoperative and intraoperative steps to achieve successful focal therapy: (1) geographically precise 3D intraprostatic localization, contouring, staging and grading of cancer lesions; (2) appropriate selection of the therapeutic technology to achieve the patient-specific goal; (3) precise intraoperative-guided ablation to ensure treatment of the targeted lesion;

(4) reliable intraoperative confirmation of destruction of the targeted cancer lesion, along with a margin of normal tissue if necessary; and (5) preservation of all uninvolved periprostatic anatomy minimizing collateral functional sequelae, optimizing QOL, and establishing a longitudinal surveillance strategy of both treated and untreated prostate tissues [27].

In the preoperative patient selection and in postoperative surveillance, reliable diagnostic or monitoring strategies are required, including (a) modern multiparametric imaging, (b) biopsy-generated data, and (c) molecular markers of various materials (serum, urine, and tissue).

For focal therapy of localized prostate cancer to be successful, we must know where the cancer is, using both imaging and documented biopsy. When the target of the index lesion is image visible, the biopsy needle as well as therapeutic probe can be guided in real time to the center of the visible lesion. This visibility would facilitate the targeted focal therapy with certain confidence in precise targeting. However, modern imaging modalities may not be accurate enough to visualize all cancer foci, as prostate cancer is often multifocal. In the case in which clinically significant cancer cannot be visualized by modern imaging modalities, another solution for achieving precise targeting is needed. This is where the three-dimensionally digitalized documentation of the biopsy-proven cancer location becomes essential. This three-dimensionally documented biopsy-site tracking is now available and will be instrumental in the future of focal therapy [17].

Visualizing and contouring a cancer lesion is the first essential step in focal therapy strategy. This allows for precise image-targeted biopsy of the center of the lesion and subsequent precise therapeutic targeting of the lesion plus margin as well as "per-lesion" follow-up on the treated lesion and "per-lesion" active surveillance of untreated lesion. Even if a random biopsy-diagnosed cancer is invisible on imaging, if that biopsy trajectory is geographically documented, we can digitally compute the 3D intraprostatic location of that biopsy-proven lesion. As such, for tissue-preserving targeted focal therapy, sophisticated imaging and/or precise geographically documented biopsies are important.

Oncological efficacy and preservation of QOL by focal therapy depend on the preoperative characterization of the prostate cancer and the ability of various emerging therapeutic modalities to ablate effectively and accurately. Selection criteria need to be determined according to the coming reports of oncological efficacy and treatment-related morbidity of each therapeutic modality. In fact, we still do not know the best energy for focal therapy of prostate cancer.

Current unresolved issues also include the lack of accurate cancer-specific predictors of tumor characterization within the context of competing risk models and the limitations associated with clinically available variables such as imaging, biopsy-generated data, and biomarkers.

Preoperative accurate localization of the cancer and intraoperative precise targeting are vital for delivering an effective focal therapy. Intraoperative TRUS guidance remains the most effective imaging modality to guide intraprostatic targeting and has been most familiar in urological practice as well as in the urological operation room. Utilization of the data of mp-MRI is now becoming crucial, which is likely achieved using recently evolved MR/US fusion techniques. In addition, new technology related with modern ultrasound technology, such as the real-time three-dimensional imagery, simultaneous biplane TRUS, US contrast enhancer, multi-planar display, various ablative energy techniques coupled with real-time US guidance, device tracking systems, and robotics, would support the several specific steps of focal therapy. When comparing the imaging between preoperative baseline and after focal therapy, the preoperatively documented signs in the biopsy-proven cancer likely disappeared, suggesting the technical success of targeted focal therapy in surveillance [28].

As better staging and characterization of the index lesion as well as possible second lesion becomes possible, focal therapy will likely be offered to a considerable proportion of prostate cancer patients. Lifetime strategy with meticulous patient selection and follow-up, in the setting of well-designed clinical studies and registries, will be necessary for successful focal therapy [1].

3.4   Transition Toward Focal Therapy for Tissue Preservation Strategy in Combination with Active Surveillance

Prior to active surveillance becoming a standard option, urologists were essentially only interested in the binary diagnosis of any cancer in the prostate in order to provide rationale for the immediate whole-gland prostate treatment. The major reason why urological surgeon offers radical surgery for patients who may be candidate of active surveillance has been mainly the sampling error of possible multifocal and/or higher-risk cancer foci in the prostate in the contemporary practice of prostate biopsy. Currently, nevertheless, patients who seek tissue preservation strategy of focal therapy are already being treated at academic and private practices, sometimes as part of Institutional Review Board-approved research, more often not [3, 29, 30].

Every effort to decrease sampling error by conventional random biopsy technique has represented a step toward focal therapy. This progress has been critical for the precise characterization and localization of prostate cancer. As recently reported, the role of prostate biopsies has changed [19]. Their importance has evolved from pure cancer detection to assisting clinical patient management.

Focal therapy is a contemporary evolution of treatment philosophy especially in light of several recent observations indicating men with prostate cancer may be underserved. Recent study by Daskivich et al. explored the relationship between age, tumor risk, and comorbid disease in the survival of men diagnosed with and treated for localized prostate cancer in the USA and revealed that the majority of patients have still undergone aggressive therapy consisting of surgery or radiation, despite many being older and/or sicker, who were much more likely to die of something other than prostate cancer [31].

Jacobs et al. looked at changes in patterns of care of low-grade prostate cancer from 2004 to 2009 in the USA and observed that the use of intensity-modulated radiotherapy and robotic surgery increased, although these newer and more expensive technologies were rapidly adopted ahead of evidence to support their superiority compared to conventional techniques [32]. However, the possible explanation for this phenomenon was suggested that there were financial incentives, including "ownership opportunities, marketing share, and reimbursement fee," that have likely driven these changes in patterns of care.

As urologists, we should learn from the recent alert of possible overtreatment of prostate cancer. We should carefully select who should be aggressively treated and who benefits from the focal therapy of prostate and/or active surveillance. It is important to acknowledge and understand the different approaches of focal therapy in which various specific selection criteria and its end points could be used. The scientific proof of the benefits for oncological and functional efficacy in each selected patients in each therapeutic modality is awaited. Importantly, the door for future era of focal therapy of prostate cancer in conjunction with active surveillance of prostate cancer is open. It should be considered objectively and examined appropriately in order to better serve men with prostate cancer.

References

1. Ward 3rd JF, Rewcastle JC, Ukimura O, Gill IS. Focal therapy for the treatment of localized prostate cancer: a potential therapeutic paradigm shift awaiting better imaging. Curr Opin Urol. 2012;22(2):104–8.
2. Eggener SE, Scardino PT, Carroll PR, Zelefsky MJ, Sartor O, Hricak H, Wheeler TM, Fine SW, Trachtenberg J, Rubin MA, Ohori M, Kuroiwa K, Rossignol M, Abenhaim L, International Task Force on Prostate Cancer and the Focal Lesion Paradigm. Focal therapy for localized prostate cancer: a critical appraisal of rationale and modalities. J Urol. 2007;178(6):2260–7.
3. Valerio M, Ahmed HU, Emberton M, Lawrentschuk N, Lazzeri M, Montironi R, Nguyen PL, Trachtenberg J, Polascik TJ. The role of focal therapy in the management of localised prostate cancer: a systematic review. Eur Urol. 2014;66:732–51.
4. Sanda MG, Dunn RL, Michalski J, Sandler HM, Northouse L, Hembroff L, Lin X, Greenfield TK, Litwin MS, Saigal CS, Mahadevan A, Klein E, Kibel A, Pisters LL, Kuban D, Kaplan I, Wood D, Ciezki J, Shah N, Wei JT. Quality of life and satisfaction with outcome among prostate-cancer survivors. N Engl J Med. 2008;358(12):1250–61.
5. Wilt TJ, Brawer MK, Jones KM, Barry MJ, Aronson WJ, Fox S, Gingrich JR, Wei JT, Gilhooly P, Grob BM, Nsouli I, Iyer P, Cartagena R, Snider G, Roehrborn C, Sharifi R, Blank W, Pandya P, Andriole GL, Culkin D, Wheeler T, Prostate Cancer Intervention versus Observation Trial (PIVOT) Study Group. Radical prostatectomy versus observation for localized prostate cancer. N Engl J Med. 2012;367(3):203–13.
6. Heidenreich A, Bastian PJ, Bellmunt J, Bolla M, Joniau S, van der Kwast T, Mason M, Matveev V, Wiegel T, Zattoni F, Mottet N. EAU guidelines on prostate cancer. Part 1: screening, diagnosis, and local treatment with curative intent-update 2013. Eur Urol. 2014;65:124–37.
7. Dall'Era MA, Albertsen PC, Bangma C, Carroll PR, Carter HB, Cooperberg MR, Freedland SJ, Klotz LH, Parker C, Soloway MS. Active surveillance for prostate cancer: a systematic review of the literature. Eur Urol. 2012;62(6):976–83.
8. Stamey TA, McNeal JM, Wise AM, Clayton JL. Secondary cancers in the prostate do not determine PSA biochemical failure in untreated men undergoing radical retropubic prostatectomy. Eur Urol. 2001;39 Suppl 4:22–3.
9. Noguchi M, Stamey TA, McNeal JE, Nolley R. Prognostic factors for multifocal prostate cancer in radical prostatectomy specimens: lack of significance of secondary cancers. J Urol. 2003;170(2 Pt 1):459–63.

10. Ahmed HU. The index lesion and the origin of prostate cancer. N Engl J Med. 2009;361(17):1704–6.
11. Cheng L, Cheville JC, Pisansky TM, Sebo TJ, Slezak J, Bergstralh EJ, Neumann RM, Singh R, Pacelli A, Zincke H, Bostwick DG. Prevalence and distribution of prostatic intraepithelial neoplasia in salvage radical prostatectomy specimens after radiation therapy. Am J Surg Pathol. 1999;23(7):803–8.
12. Wallace T, Avital I, Stojadinovic A, Brücher BL, Cote E, Yu J. Multi-parametric MRI-directed focal salvage permanent interstitial brachytherapy for locally recurrent adenocarcinoma of the prostate: a novel approach. J Cancer. 2013;4(2):146–51.
13. Sidana A, Chowdhury WH, Fuchs EJ, Rodriguez R. Cryoimmunotherapy in urologic oncology. Urology. 2010;75(5):1009–14.
14. Waitz R, Solomon SB, Petre EN, Trumble AE, Fassò M, Norton L, Allison JP. Potent induction of tumor immunity by combining tumor cryoablation with anti-CTLA-4 therapy. Cancer Res. 2012;72(2):430–9.
15. Xia JZ, Xie FL, Ran LF, Xie XP, Fan YM, Wu F. High-intensity focused ultrasound tumor ablation activates autologous tumor-specific cytotoxic T lymphocytes. Ultrasound Med Biol. 2012;38(8):1363–71.
16. Ukimura O. Image-guided surgery in minimally invasive urology. Curr Opin Urol. 2010;20:136–40.
17. Ukimura O, Hung A, Gill IS. Innovations in prostate biopsy strategies for active surveillance and focal therapy. Curr Opin Urol. 2011;21:115–20.
18. Onik G, Miessau M, Bostwick DG. Three-dimensional prostate mapping biopsy has a potentially significant impact on prostate cancer management. J Clin Oncol. 2009;27:4321–6.
19. Ukimura O, Coleman J, de la Taille A, Emberton M, Epstein J, Freedland S, Giannarini G, Kibel A, Montironi R, Ploussard G, Roobol M, Scattoni V, Jones S. Contemporary role of systematic prostate biopsies: indications, technique, implications on patient care. Eur Urol. 2013;63(2):214–30.
20. Moore CM, Robertosn NL, Arsanious N, et al. Image-guided prostate biopsy using magnetic resonance imaging–derived targets: a systematic review. Eur Urol. 2013;63:125–40.
21. Ukimura O, Abreu AL, Gill IS, Shoji S, Hung AJ, Bahn D. Image-visibility of cancer to enhance targeting precision and spatial mapping biopsy for focal therapy of prostate cancer. BJU Int. 2013;111(8):E354–64.
22. Ukimura O, Troncoso P, Ramirez EI, Babaian RJ. Prostate cancer staging: correlation between ultrasound determined tumor contact length and pathologically confirmed extraprostatic extension. J Urol. 1998;159:1251–9.
23. Mazaheri Y, Hricak H, Fine SW, Akin O, Shukla-Dave A, Ishill NM, Moskowitz CS, Grater JE, Reuter VE, Zakian KL, Touijer KA, Koutcher JA. Prostate tumor volume measurement with combined T2-weighted imaging and diffusion-weighted MR: correlation with pathologic tumor volume. Radiology. 2009;252(2):449–57.
24. Turkbey B, Mani H, Aras O, Rastinehad AR, Shah V, Bernardo M, Pohida T, Daar D, Benjamin C, McKinney YL, Linehan WM, Wood BJ, Merino MJ, Choyke PL, Pinto PA. Correlation of magnetic resonance imaging tumor volume with histopathology. J Urol. 2012;188(4):1157–63.
25. Tanaka K, Shigemura K, Muramaki M, Takahashi S, Miyake H, Fujisawa M. Efficacy of using three-tesla magnetic resonance imaging diagnosis of capsule invasion for decision-making about neurovascular bundle preservation in robotic-assisted radical prostatectomy. Korean J Urol. 2013;54(7):437–41.
26. Hwii Ko Y, Jae Sung D, Gu Kang S, Ho Kang S, Gu Lee J, Jong Kim J, Cheon J. The predictability of T3 disease in staging MRI following prostate biopsy decreases in patients with high initial PSA and Gleason score. Asian J Androl. 2011;13(3):487–93.
27. Ukimura O, Gill IS. Editorials: key to successful focal therapy: location, location. Location Eur Urol. 2012;62(1):66–7.
28. Ukimura O, Faber K, Gill IS. Intra-prostatic targeting. Curr Opin Urol. 2012;22:97–103.

29. Bahn D, de Castro Abreu AL, Gill IS, Hung AJ, Silverman P, Gross ME, Lieskovsky G, Ukimura O. Focal cryotherapy for clinically unilateral low-intermediate risk prostate cancer in 73 men with median 3.7-year follow-up. Eur Urol. 2012;62(1):55–63.
30. Ahmed HU, Hindley RG, Dickinson L, Freeman A, Kirkham AP, Sahu M, Scott R, Allen C, Van der Meulen J, Emberton M. Focal therapy for localised unifocal and multifocal prostate cancer: a prospective development study. Lancet Oncol. 2012;13(6):622–32.
31. Daskivich TJ, Fan KH, Koyama T, Albertsen PC, Goodman M, Hamilton AS, Hoffman RM, Stanford JL, Stroup AM, Litwin MS, Penson DF. Effect of age, tumor risk, and comorbidity on competing risks for survival in a U.S. population-based cohort of men with prostate cancer. Ann Intern Med. 2013;158(10):709–17.
32. Jacobs BL, Zhang Y, Schroeck FR, Skolarus TA, Wei JT, Montie JE, Gilbert SM, Strope SA, Dunn RL, Miller DC, Hollenbeck BK. Use of advanced treatment technologies among men at low risk of dying from prostate cancer. JAMA. 2013;309(24):2587–95.

Part II
New Diagnostics

How Do We Select Patients Eligible for Focal Therapy? Imaging and Targeted Biopsies: A Basic Prerequisite for Focal Therapy

4

Eduard Baco, Viktor Berge, and Erik Rud

Contents

Aims of this chapter are to highlight the following:

- The concept of significant and insignificant cancer
- The importance of identifying the index tumor
- Benefits and limitations of MRI
- Optimal biopsy strategy

E. Baco (✉) • V. Berge
Department of Urology, Oslo University Hospital, Oslo, Norway
e-mail: BACE@ous-hf.no; vikber@ous-hf.no

E. Rud
Department of Radiology, Oslo University Hospital, Oslo, Norway
e-mail: p.e.rud@medisin.uio.no

© Springer International Publishing Switzerland 2015
S. Thüroff, C.G. Chaussy (eds.), *Focal Therapy of Prostate Cancer:*
An Emerging Strategy for Minimally Invasive, Staged Treatment,
DOI 10.1007/978-3-319-14160-2_4

4.1   Introduction

Focal therapy for prostate cancer has been increasingly utilized with the goal of effective disease control while maximizing patient functional outcomes. Potential drawbacks include the risk of incomplete treatment, which may result from missed clinical significant cancer foci and inadequate ablation to target tissues.

The optimal selection criteria for focal therapy are not known and therefore not standardized. In a recent international multidisciplinary consensus meeting, chaired by Dr. Peter Scardino, the following inclusion criteria were recommended [1]:

- PSA < 15 ng/ml. Patients with PSA > 15 ng/ml should be counseled with caution.
- Clinical stage T1c-T2a.
- Pathology GS ≤ 3 + 4.

4.2   Index Tumor and Clinical Significant Disease

In case of multifocal prostate cancer, there is increasing evidence that the largest tumor (the index tumor) drives the natural history of prostate cancer [2]. The clinical importance of identifying the index tumor is related to the close association with extraprostatic extension (EPE) and the highest GS [3].

Is unifocal disease the sine qua non for focal prostate therapy? Pathological data support the concept that small-volume, low-grade tumors do not worsen the prognosis, and consequently one could treat the index tumor and leave the secondary non-clinical significant tumor foci for surveillance [3]. Current criteria for insignificant prostate cancer in radical prostatectomy (RP) specimens include organ-confined cancer, absence of Gleason grade 4/5, or maximum tumor volume (TV) of 0.5 ml [4].

Rud et al. [5] demonstrated that MRI detected 92 % of all index tumors and 86 % of all tumors >0.5 ml. However, 22 % had undetected secondary tumors with GS 7 or higher, although the volumes were all <0.4 ml.

Since MRI cannot detect all significant tumors, how can we rule out the invisible tumors in patients planned for focal therapy?

4.3   Accuracy of mpMRI in Detecting the Index Tumor and Assessing TV

- MRI is the best tool for detecting the index tumor.
- Using MRI for estimation of TV is subject to controversy, and caution is recommended when included in patient management.

The clinical concept of the index tumor is quite new, and very few MRI studies have reported the index tumor detection rates. Virtually all studies prior to 2013 focused upon the overall detection rates, often stratified according to pathological

TV. Furthermore, few studies have compared MRI and pathological TV, and only two studies are available for comparison [5, 6]. These studies reported 92 and 94 % sensitivity for detecting the index tumor. One reported no difference in TV, while the other underestimated the MRI TV compared to pathological TV. Rud et al. also used a 30-sector tumor map to assess the overall tumor burden. They demonstrated only 50 % rate of true tumor-positive sectors and 88 % true tumor-negative sectors. This finding also indicates significantly underestimation of tumor burden.

Using MRI to estimate TV is subject to controversy because it is not clear which sequences to use. Furthermore, it is not clear which volume formula to use. A typical tumor has a dense center and several extensions in different directions. For these reasons, it is not universally accepted how to measure TV on neither MRI nor pathological examination. Several suggestions have been proposed, including spherical or ellipsoid TV or the longest tumor diameter. However, none of these formulas reflect the true TV, and a planimetric examination is regarded as the most accurate method, although not feasible in a routine clinical setting. Perera et al. demonstrated that the ellipsoid volume formula generated the closest match to the planimetric reference value [7]. A consensus meeting arranged by the Society of Urogenital Pathologists in 2011 agreed that the three longest perpendicular diameters and the longest tumor diameter should be reported when assessing the whole-mounted histological examination [8].

4.4 How Should the MRI Be Performed? Which Functional Parameters Are Necessary?

- It is sufficient to only include T2 and DWI for tumor detection.
- High Gleason score (GS) is associated with restricted diffusion.
- MRI provides high negative predictive values (NPV) in low-risk groups for predicting pT3.

There is controversy regarding how and when to perform the MRI examination.

When radiologists started to use MRI in the 1990s, only anatomical T1 and T2 images were available, and the initial performance was poor compared to the current standard. Later on, functional sequences revolutionized tumor detection rates. The first important improvement was due to dynamic contrast-enhanced (DCE) MRI. Later on, diffusion-weighted images (DWI) and MR spectroscopy (MRS) were introduced. At the same time, stronger magnetic fields and better coils were developed. There is no evidence that 3 T magnetic field improves neither detection nor staging compared to 1.5 T. Furthermore, there is no evidence that an endorectal coil improves detection compared to surface coils.

4.4.1 Tumor Detection

The typical feature of a tumor on MRI is homogeneous low T2 signal and restricted diffusion.

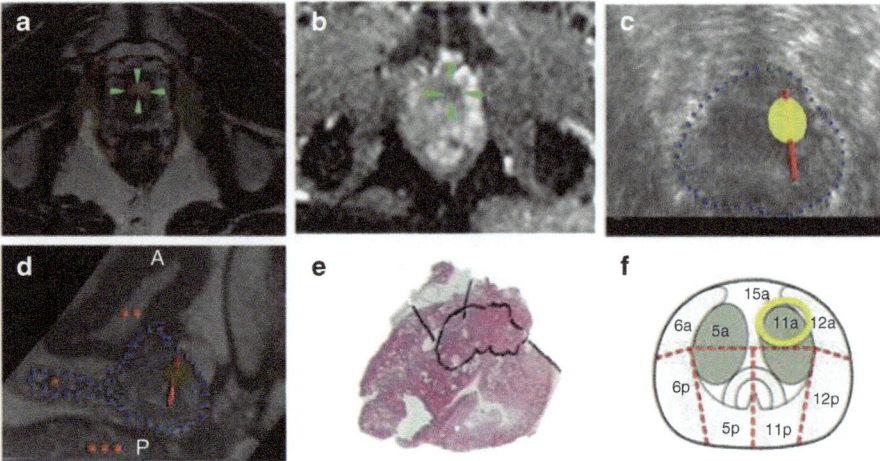

Fig. 4.1 Images for a 64-year-old man with PSA 20 ng/ml, prostate volume 67 ml, and a normal DRE previously underwent three negative random Bx procedures. (**a**) T2-corrected b-max prostate MRI and (**b**) ADC map (*green arrows*) suggested anterior tumor in the apex. Subsequent MR-TRUS cognitive fused Bx combined with random sampling showed clinically insignificant Pca GS 6 (3+3) with 2.5 mm cancer length. The fifth Bx procedure was done by MR-TRUS elastic fusion (*red bar*) and revealed Pca GS 7b (4+3) with core cancer length 13 mm (93 % core). Histological analyses of whole-gland step-sectioned prostate showed pT3a Pca GS 7a (3+4). The spatial distribution of targeted biopsy (*red bar*) and targeted region (*yellow circle*) in axial (**c**) and sagittal views (**d**) corresponded with 3D tumor location in segment 11a. (**e**) histological analysis of whole gland step-sectioned prostate showed pT3 PCa GS 7a (3+4). (**f, d**) MR-TRUS fused prostate image in sagittal view, where *** rectum, ** bladder, * vesicula seminalis

Restricted diffusion is indicated by a low apparent diffusion coefficient (ADC), which is known to inversely correlate with GS. In other words, higher GS features lower ADC. The typical feature of cancer in the DWI and ADC map is high signal on high b-value images and low signal in the ADC map. However, the absolute ADC values are highly dependent on several external factors, such as size of regions of interest, magnetic field, b-values, and time of repetition. For these reasons, caution should be addressed when measuring the ADC values in a daily clinical practice. Despite its limitations, the ADC map is probably the most important tool for identifying the area with the highest GS.

In 2012, the European Society of Urogenital Radiology (ESUR) recommended including T2, DCE, and DWI, while MRS was not included [9]. T2 is needed for anatomy and for better evaluating tumors in the transition zone. Many regard DCE to be important for improving the sensitivity, while DWI improves the specificity. However, no studies have shown that DCE improves the sensitivity compared to DWI, and today T2 and DWI seem sufficient for tumor detection [10]. Different post-processing tools are also available and may help in improving tumor detection further. These softwares help to remove unwanted "noise" in the image and highlight features known to characterize a tumor (Figs. 4.1 and 4.2). A standardized scoring system (Pi-RAD 1-5) has been developed, and >3 indicates that significant cancer is likely.

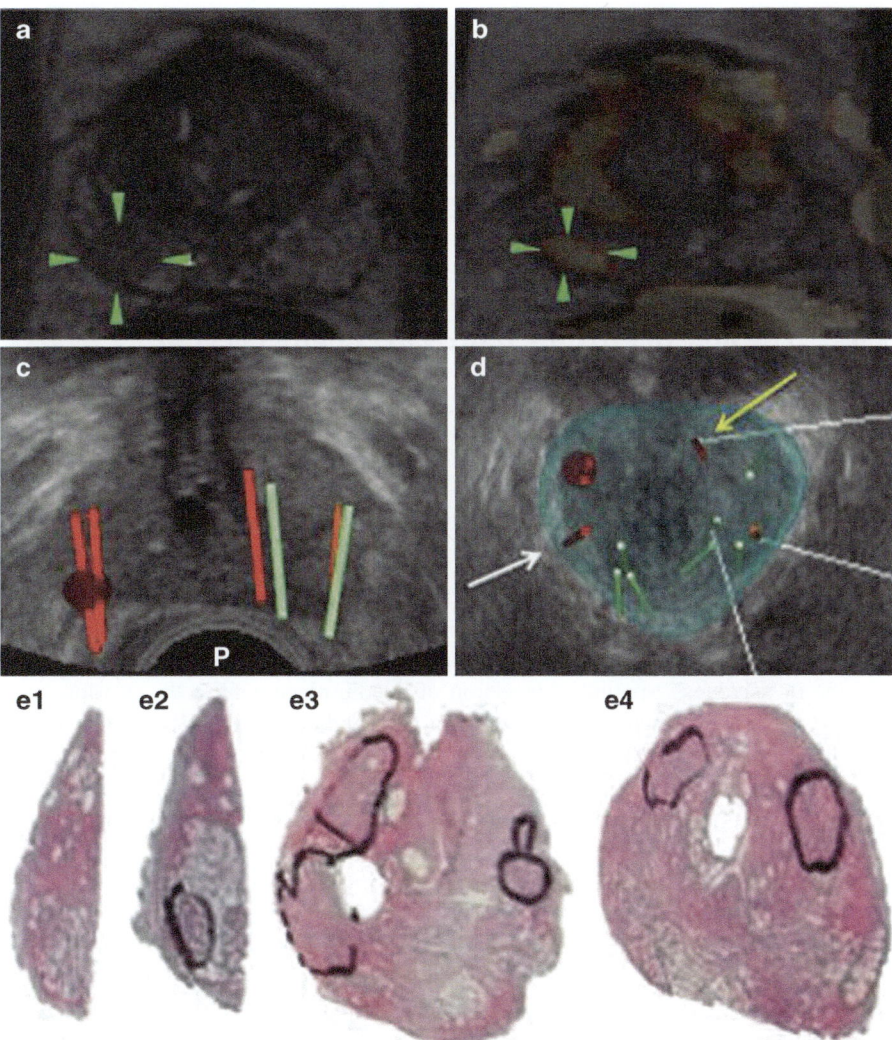

Fig. 4.2 Images for a 59-year-old man with PSA 4.0 ng/ml and normal DRE. (**a**) T2-weighted MRI and (**b**) T2-corrected b-max axial MRI suggest a solitary, highly suspicious tumor with diameter 10 mm localized in the right base (*green arrows*). (**c**) Axial real-time MR/US fusion image shows the suspicious tumor marked as a *red circle*. Two *red bars* in this circle represent two targeted biopsies. Histology revealed Pca GS 7 (3+4) with cancer core length 10 and 3 mm. (**d**) Coronal real-time fusion image shows the spatial distribution of all biopsies. One of random biopsies in the right prostate lobe (*red bar* marked with *white arrow*) identified Pca GS 6 (3+3) with cancer core length 8 mm. Another random biopsy in the left base (*red bar* marked with *yellow arrow*) revealed Pca GS 8 (4+4) with cancer core length 3 mm. *Green bars* represent negative biopsies. This patient was not suitable for focal therapy and was treated by radical prostatectomy. (**e1–4**) Histological analyses of step-sectioned prostate concluded with pT2c Pca GS 7 (3+4), diameters 13×10×10 mm and 15×8×8 mm localized in the left prostate lobe. Right prostate base harbored Pca GS 3+4, diameter 10×5×5 mm. This tumor was MRI invisible. The spatial distribution of positive random biopsies corresponded with location and extension of index tumor and secondary cancer foci

4.4.2 MRI and T Classification

MRI offers limited sensitivity for detecting extraprostatic (pT3) disease in unselected patient cohorts. A recent study demonstrated 73 % sensitivity and 58 % specificity for predicting pT3 [11]. In the low- and intermediary-risk group, 88 and 57 % negative predictive values were found, respectively. In other words, there is substantial risk for wrongfully recommending FT to intermediate-risk patients who might have extraprostatic extension.

4.5 The Role of Prostate Biopsy in Patient Selection to Focal Therapy

The primary challenge in patient selection to focal therapy (FT) is assessment of the cancer location, TV, and GS.

There have been long discussions about optimal prostate biopsy technique before FT. Previous studies have demonstrated that traditional transrectal ultrasound (TRUS)-guided 12-core prostate biopsy (Bx) cannot reliably predict location and extent of prostate cancer [12]. Transperineal template prostate-mapping (TTPM) biopsy was consequently accepted as the most optimal strategy for selection to FT [13]. However, this approach has several serious drawbacks, the most important include invasiveness, spatial imprecision of needle placement in the prostate, elevated risk for overdetection of insignificant foci, and cost of the procedure.

The role of prostate biopsy in selection of patients to FT is challenging and is more complex than simple cancer identification [14]. Firstly, biopsy has to confirm the MRI findings and tumor extension. Evaluation of cancer invasion in the extreme apex, seminal vesicles, and capsule may be difficult on MRI. Thus, merging of image-documented biopsy data with MRI findings may improve the pretreatment staging. Secondly, it is known that MRI frequently underestimates the histopathological TV. Adding the length of cancer involvement on targeted biopsy to MRI measurements may potentially enhance the precision of the TV estimation. Thirdly, accurate GS on biopsy is important for treatment decision-making. MRI/TRUS-targeted biopsy (TB) demonstrated high GS concordance in correlation with radical prostatectomy specimen [15].

The prostate biopsy strategy should correspond to the purpose of the treatment.

Protocols used in FT have two different ambitions: The first approach aims to perform ablation of the index tumor including the peritumoral tissue. The challenging issue is how wide peritumoral margin has to be. Functional outcomes and side effects of FT depend on the energy volume used in proximity of critical periprostatic structures. The negative biopsies in the apex and near prostate capsule may advocate for apex-sparing and nerve-sparing treatments. Our results have demonstrated that apex-sparing salvage HIFU preserves the continence in patients with radiorecurrent prostate cancer [16]. The irritative urinary symptoms, which frequently occur after whole-gland ablation, may be avoided or shortened by bladder neck and/or urethra-sparing procedure.

The second FT approach known as hemi-ablation of the prostate aims to completely eradicate the cancer in one lobe. In this approach, the regular distribution of Bx cores in non-treated lobe will improve the quality of biopsy sampling and reduce the chance to miss significant cancer.

4.6   Targeted Prostate Biopsy

Targeted biopsy (TB) of MRI-suspected abnormalities has been a common practice before inclusion of patient to FT. There are different ways for performing targeted biopsy procedure.

The MRI radiologists can perform the biopsy of suspicious regions within the MR scanner [17]. The major concern of this "in-bore" biopsy is that the patient has to undergo two separate MRI sessions. The biopsy procedure time is longer than the time needed for image acquisition. In an era where overall MRI capacity is reduced and the demand for TB is growing, it was important to find "out-bore" modalities to perform TB. Actually three different categories of targeting exist [18]:

(a) *Cognitive (visual) targeting* which depends on the physician's capability to visually estimate the MR suspicious area in the TRUS image at the time of Bx [19]. It is important to keep in mind that the urologist and radiologist probably have different opinions about where the boundaries of the different regions are. Consequently, it is difficult for the urologist to perform an accurate targeted biopsy based on a written paper alone.
(b) *Sensor-based registration* where a "rigid" fusion of MR and TRUS images is performed by a software followed by tracking of the US probe by magnetic sensor. However, it does not take into account the prostate deformation and prostate movement during the procedure [20, 21].
(c) *Organ-based elastic MRI/TRUS image fusion* that factors in consideration of the prostate and patient movements, both during the initial fusion and planning and during the organ tracking phase at the time of Bx [22].

4.7   The Precision of the Different Fusion Systems

The diagnostic performance of visual and rigid fusion has been evaluated in two prospective studies where different rigid fused systems were used. No significant difference in cancer detection rate (CDR) between the fusion modalities was found [19, 23]. It is important to note that experts in this field performed visual TB. The authors conclude that the use of an image fusion platform may be beneficial for targeting smaller tumor as well as for the urologists with limited experience in the field of MRI and visual targeting.

CDR of visual, rigid, and elastic fusion in initial Bx setting was evaluated in a large prospective study [24]. The results have demonstrated a significantly higher CDR for clinically significant cancers using elastic fusion.

The accuracy of elastic MRI/TRUS fusion in index tumor diagnostics was recently evaluated in clinical two-centered study which carried 110 patients [15]. MRI and TB results were correlated with pathological findings on step-sectioned RP specimens. The results demonstrated that TB can reliably (≥90 %) predict location and primary Gleason grade pattern of the index tumor with relatively limited estimation of index tumor volume and overall GS. Only 2 cores per index tumor were performed for achieving the diagnosis (Fig. 4.1).

4.8   Clinical Workup of Elastic MRI/TRUS Image Fusion-Guided Targeted Biopsy

TB performed using elastic fusion is a complex procedure where five consecutive steps are applied: (1) identification of the suspicious region in pre-biopsy MRI, (2) online transferring of 3D MRI volume data to workstation, (3) acquisition of real-time 3D-TRUS of the prostate, (4) MR-TRUS elastic image fusion, and (5) TB of MRI suspicious regions with digitalized documentation of each biopsy trajectory [25].

The key of precision of this targeted procedure is based on automatic, nonrigid (elastic) registration technology [26]. The physician performing the biopsy maintains the biopsy needle after firing in prostate for approximately 3 s. During this time, real-time 3D-TRUS acquisitions are repeated, and biopsy trajectory is automatically documented by software in 3D volume data of the prostate. The biopsy procedure is free hand based and could be performed with local anesthesia in an outpatient clinic.

4.9   What Is the Role of Systematic Prostate Biopsy and How Can We Rule Out Invisible Tumors?

As mentioned in the imaging chapter, MRI is the most precise imaging tool for diagnosing Pca. However, nonspecific MRI findings are frequent and need to be clarified by biopsy. Further, MRI cannot identify all clinically significant tumors, especially if density of tumor tissue is low.

Traditional TRUS-guided random Bx is regularly performed using two-plan ultrasound guidance. The major shortcoming of this technique is that the accurate biopsy needle position in the prostate cannot be documented. In case of positive biopsy results, precise interpretation of location and extension of cancer tissue is difficult.

A computerized 3D-TRUS system is equipped with automatic registration of each biopsy trajectory in 3D prostate volume. The biopsy trajectory is visible in real time during the biopsy procedure and allows for performing organized distribution of biopsy cores in all prostate segments. Using navigation technology, all prostate regions can be sampled [27].

Due to mentioned limitations of MRI, the systematic biopsy procedures before FT still have importance. However, the optimal quantity of biopsy cores and their geographical distribution are debated. In candidates to FT, we first perform TB using 1–2 cores per each MRI visible abnormality. Then we perform systematic prostate mapping by 12 biopsy cores. Navigation system and superimposed grid help to localize the biopsy centrally in each prostate sextant. The accuracy of biopsy distribution is based on organ tracking and image-registered localization of each core.

We believe that a systematic core distribution may limit sampling error and consequently reduce the risk for missing significant tumors. Contrary to saturation biopsy procedure, this 12-core organized mapping may reduce the chance for over-detection of micro-focal cancers. Nevertheless, the reliability of this method in patient selection for FT needs to be evaluated by prospective studies.

A digitally stored 3D registration of biopsy locations has importance for evaluation of cancer extension. Each biopsy trajectory can be revisualized after histological analyses are completed. If necessary, the specific prostate area could be retargeted, and/or additional biopsies could be localized in the previously unsampled regions. Displayed biopsy cartography on computer screen or in PDF file can be discussed with the patients and their family during decision-making and consent focal therapy planning (Fig. 4.2).

References

1. van den Bos W, Muller BG, Ahmed H, Bangma CH, Barret E, Crouzet S, et al. Focal therapy in prostate cancer: international multidisciplinary consensus on trial design. Eur Urol. 2014;13.
2. Ahmed HU. The index lesion and the origin of prostate cancer. N Engl J Med. 2009; 361(17):1704–6.
3. Bostwick DG, Waters DJ, Farley ER, Meiers I, Rukstalis D, Cavanaugh WA, et al. Group consensus reports from the Consensus Conference on Focal Treatment of Prostatic Carcinoma, Celebration, Florida, February 24, 2006. Urology. 2007;70(6 Suppl):42–4.
4. Epstein JI, Walsh PC, Carmichael M, Brendler CB. Pathologic and clinical findings to predict tumor extent of nonpalpable (stage T1c) prostate cancer. JAMA. 1994;271(5):368–74.
5. Rud E, Klotz D, Rennesund K, Baco E, Berge V, Lien D, et al. Detection of the Index Tumor and Tumor Volume in Prostate Cancer using T2w and DW MRI alone. BJU Int. 2014;21.
6. Turkbey B, Mani H, Aras O, Rastinehad AR, Shah V, Bernardo M, et al. Correlation of magnetic resonance imaging tumor volume with histopathology. J Urol. 2012;188(4):1157–63.
7. Perera M, Lawrentschuk N, Bolton D, Clouston D. Comparison contemporary methods of estimating prostate tumor volume in pathological specimens. BJU Int. 2013;113 Suppl 2: 29–34.
8. van der Kwast TH, Amin MB, Billis A, Epstein JI, Griffiths D, Humphrey PA, et al. International Society of Urological Pathology (ISUP) Consensus Conference on Handling and Staging of Radical Prostatectomy Specimens. Working group 2: T2 substaging and prostate cancer volume. Mod Pathol. 2010;24(1):16–25. Nature Publishing Group.
9. Barentsz JO, Richenberg J, Clements R, Choyke P, Verma S, Villeirs G, et al. ESUR prostate MR guidelines 2012. Eur Radiol. 2012;22(4):746–57.
10. Haghighi M, Shah S, Taneja SS, Rosenkrantz AB. Prostate cancer: diffusion-weighted imaging versus dynamic-contrast enhanced imaging for tumor localization-a meta-analysis. J Comput Assist Tomogr. 2013;37(6):980–8.

11. Somford DM, Hamoen EH, Fütterer JJ, van Basten JP, Hulsbergen-Van de Kaa CA, Vreuls W, et al. The predictive value of endorectal 3 tesla multiparametric magnetic resonance imaging for extraprostatic extension in patients with low, intermediate and high risk prostate cancer. J Urol. 2013;190(5):1728–34.

12. Washington SL, Bonham M, Whitson JM, Cowan JE, Carroll PR. Transrectal ultrasonography-guided biopsy does not reliably identify dominant cancer location in men with low-risk prostate cancer. BJU Int [Internet]. 2011;110(1):50–5.

13. Singh PB, Anele C, Dalton E, Barbouti O, Stevens D, Gurung P, et al. Prostate cancer tumour features on template prostate-mapping biopsies: implications for focal therapy. Eur Urol. 2014 Jul;66(1):12–9 Available from: http://dx.doi.org/10.1016/j.eururo.2013.09.045.

14. Ukimura O, Gill IS. Targeted prostate biopsies for a histogram of the index lesion. Curr Opin Urol [Internet]. 2013;23(2):118–22.

15. Berge V, Baco E, Karlsen SJ. A prospective study of salvage high-intensity focused ultrasound for locally radiorecurrent prostate cancer: early results. Scand J Urol Nephrol. 2010;44(4):223–7.

16. Berge V, Baco E, Dahl AA, Karlsen SJ. Health-related quality of life after salvage high-intensity focused ultrasound (HIFU) treatment for locally radiorecurrent prostate cancer. Int J Urol [Internet]. 2011;18(9):646–51. Available from: http://www.ncbi.nlm.nih.gov/pubmed/21771102.

17. Hoeks CMA, Schouten MG, Bomers JGR, Hoogendoorn SP, Hulsbergen-Van de Kaa CA, Hambrock T, et al. Three-tesla magnetic resonance-guided prostate biopsy in men with increased prostate-specific antigen and repeated, negative, random, systematic, transrectal ultrasound biopsies: detection of clinically significant prostate cancers. Eur Urol. 2012; 62(5):902–9.

18. Cornud F, Brolis L, Delongchamps NB, Portalez D, Malavaud B, Renard-Penna R, et al. TRUS–MRI image registration: a paradigm shift in the diagnosis of significant prostate cancer. Abdom Imaging [Internet]. 2013;38(6):1447–63. Available from: http://link.springer.com/10.1007/s00261-013-0018-4.

19. Puech P, Rouvière O, Renard-Penna R, Villers A, Devos P, Colombel M, et al. Prostate cancer diagnosis: multiparametric MR-targeted biopsy with cognitive and transrectal US-MR fusion guidance versus systematic biopsy – prospective multicenter study. Radiology [Internet]. 2013;268(2):461–9. Available from: http://www.ncbi.nlm.nih.gov/pubmed/23579051

20. Pinto PA, Chung PH, Rastinehad AR, Baccala Jr AA, Kruecker J, Benjamin CJ, et al. Magnetic resonance imaging/ultrasound fusion guided prostate biopsy improves cancer detection following transrectal ultrasound biopsy and correlates with multiparametric magnetic resonance imaging. J Urol. 2011;186(4):1281–5. American Urological Association Education and Research, Inc.

21. Siddiqui MM, Rais-Bahrami S, Truong H, Stamatakis L, Vourganti S, Nix J, et al. Magnetic resonance imaging/ultrasound–fusion biopsy significantly upgrades prostate cancer versus systematic 12-core transrectal ultrasound biopsy. Eur Urol [Internet]. 2013;64(5):713–9. Available from: http://dx.doi.org/10.1016/j.eururo.2013.05.059. European Association of Urology.

22. Rud E, Baco E, Eggesbø HB. MRI and ultrasound-guided prostate biopsy using soft image fusion. Anticancer Res. 2012;32(8):3383–9.

23. Wysock JS, Rosenkrantz AB, Huang WC, Stifelman MD, Lepor H, Deng F-M, et al. A prospective, blinded comparison of magnetic resonance (MR) imaging–ultrasound fusion and visual estimation in the performance of MR-targeted prostate biopsy: The PROFUS Trial. Eur Urol. 2014 Aug;66(2):343–51 Available from: http://dx.doi.org/10.1016/j.eururo.2013.10.048. European Association of Urology.

24. Delongchamps NB, Peyromaure M, Schull A, Beuvon F, Bouazza N, Flam T, et al. Pre-biopsy magnetic resonance imaging and prostate cancer detection: comparison of random and MRI-targeted biopsies using three different techniques of MRI-TRUS image registration. J Urol. 2012;13.

25. Portalez D, Mozer P, Cornud F, Renard-Penna R, Misrai V, Thoulouzan M, et al. Validation of the European Society of Urogenital Radiology scoring system for prostate cancer diagnosis on multiparametric magnetic resonance imaging in a cohort of repeat biopsy patients. Eur Urol [Internet]. 2012;62(6):986–96.
26. Baumann M, Mozer P, Daanen V, Troccaz J. Prostate biopsy tracking with deformation estimation. Med Image Anal. 2011;16(3):562–76.
27. Ukimura O, Desai MM, Palmer S, Valencerina S, Gross M, Abreu AL, et al. 3-Dimensional elastic registration system of prostate biopsy location by real-time 3-dimensional transrectal ultrasound guidance with magnetic resonance/transrectal ultrasound image fusion. J Urol [Internet]. 2012;187(3):1080–6. Available from: http://dx.doi.org/10.1016/j.juro.2011.10.124. Elsevier Inc.

"How to Make TRUS Better": HistoScanning-Guided Biopsies for Identification of Cancer Within the Prostate

5

Moritz F. Hamann and Klaus-Peter Jünemann

Contents

5.1   Introduction

In contrast to most other imaging tools, transrectal ultrasound of the prostate (TRUS) has the unique advantages of infinite access, portability, real-time imaging, low cost, and ease of use. TRUS technique reliably visualizes zonal anatomy, volume, and benign as well as malignant prostatic lesions like prostate carcinoma, which typically presents as hypoechoic areas within the peripheral zone. But accurate picture interpretation requires comprehensive expertise and inevitably includes a high interobserver variability. Furthermore, hypoechoic gray-scale patterns in B-mode TRUS are not highly sensitive or specific for the detection of prostate carcinoma [7]. In summary, TRUS imaging does not achieve up-to-date requirements like standardization, examiner independency, and high diagnostic accuracy as a key challenge for modern/future prostate cancer therapy.

M.F. Hamann (✉) • K.-P. Jünemann
Kiel, Germany
e-mail: moritz.hamann@uksh.de

© Springer International Publishing Switzerland 2015
S. Thüroff, C.G. Chaussy (eds.), *Focal Therapy of Prostate Cancer:*
An Emerging Strategy for Minimally Invasive, Staged Treatment,
DOI 10.1007/978-3-319-14160-2_5

51

Multiple approaches including contrast-enhanced transrectal ultrasound (CE-TRUS), real-time elastography (RTE), or computerized transrectal ultrasound (C-TRUS) have been shown to reduce technical limitations and to aid in diagnosis of prostate cancer by improving delineation of abnormal tissue. They have found that targeted biopsies obtained with augmented TRUS modalities are more likely to reveal prostate cancers compared to the systematic prostate biopsy [1, 4, 10]. Another strategy for improving prostate cancer risk stratification is the use of prostate HistoScanning™ (Advanced Medical Diagnostics, Waterloo BE), an ultrasound-based tissue characterization application [2, 3]. HistoScanning analysis uses three-dimensional (3D) ultrasound data collected from a clinical TRUS examination to visualize and locate tissues suspected of harboring prostate cancer.

5.2   The Basic Principle and Analysis Algorithms of HistoScanning™

TRUS images are acquired by sending out an ultrasonic pulse into the prostate. The scanner tracks the wave front and records the signals echoing from tissue boundaries (Fig. 5.1). In conventional B-mode imaging, which displays the macroscopic features of the organ, the brightness of each point in the image represents the intensity of the echo from a particular location in the prostate. However, the reflected signals not only contain echoes from macroscopic tissue boundaries, but also a continuous stream of echoes emanating from microscopic features and histological structure of the prostatic tissue, known as ultrasound backscatter (Fig. 5.2). In conventional B-mode gray-scale imaging, ultrasound backscatter is often filtered out to create a more appealing image. While the resolution of the backscatter image is not sufficient to determine the precise prostate histology, the unfiltered backscattered information contains a signature of the tissue's underlying microstructures. The ultrasound backscatter properties of malignant or other suspicious tissues vary from that of normal prostatic tissue due to differences in, e.g., the abnormal tissue stiffness, irregular growth patterns, and invasion into blood or lymphatic vessels.

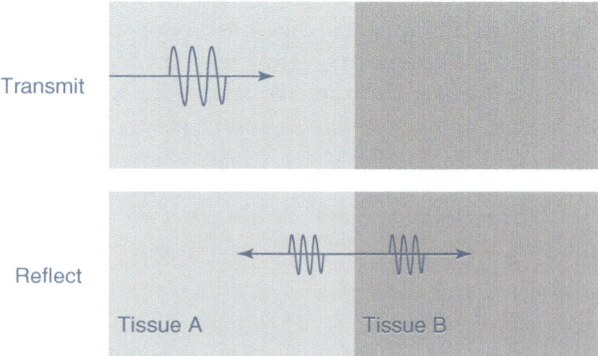

Fig. 5.1 Model of a reflection of an acoustic wave at a tissue boundary

Fig. 5.2 Model of scattered reflections (backscatter) in small-scale heterogeneous media

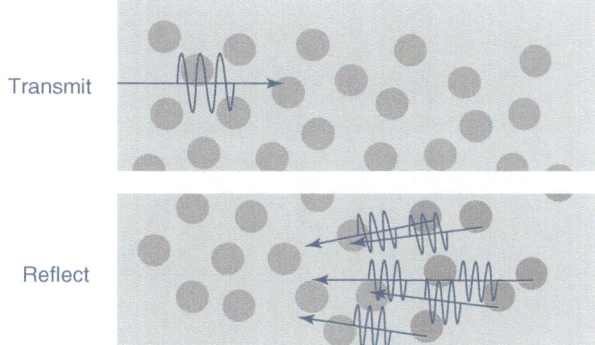

Displaying the information of ultrasound backscatter properties complements the conventional ultrasound gray-scale imaging significantly.

HistoScanning analysis requires a continuous set of 3D ultrasound data including the raw or native radio-frequency (RF) signals acquired from a high-resolution ultrasound scanner. To facilitate appropriate data acquisition and standardized scanning process, an external motor sweeps the ultrasound probe's sagittal array. After the definition of volume of interest, the HistoScanning algorithm divides the corresponding 3D raw data into small sub-volumes called tagged units (typically 7,000, depending on the size of the prostate). Each tagged unit is individually characterized using numerical descriptors of multiparametric ultrasound backscatter measures of tissue, e.g., density and homogeneity of acoustical scatterers and irregular/unusual patterns of scattering. Finally, a statistical classifier categorizes individual tagged units as normal or suspicious. Results are shown as a colored (red) overlay in the visualization volume displayed to the user (Fig. 5.3). Parallel, a second algorithm identifies low-quality data, e.g., due to shadows cast by calcifications, and displays the volumes to the user as differently colored (purple) overlays. Finally, HistoScanning provides a quasi-3D visualization or a transversal slice report of the prostate with suspicious areas highlighted (Fig. 5.4). Based on these HistoScanning images, the physician is able to define and locate target regions within the prostate. The 3D metrical report allows stereotactical guidance of perineal prostate biopsy procedures.

5.3   Transrectal HistoScanning Targeted Biopsy

With HistoScanning TT (true targeting, TT), an additional software tool, the operator is able to define specific locations within the 3D visualization volume for targeting. HistoScanning TT then provides visual feedback and instruction (rotate, tilt, and translate) using overlays of prostate boundaries fused with real-time TRUS. This allows the operator to position the transducer fitted with needle guide so that the sample core intersects with the selected target.

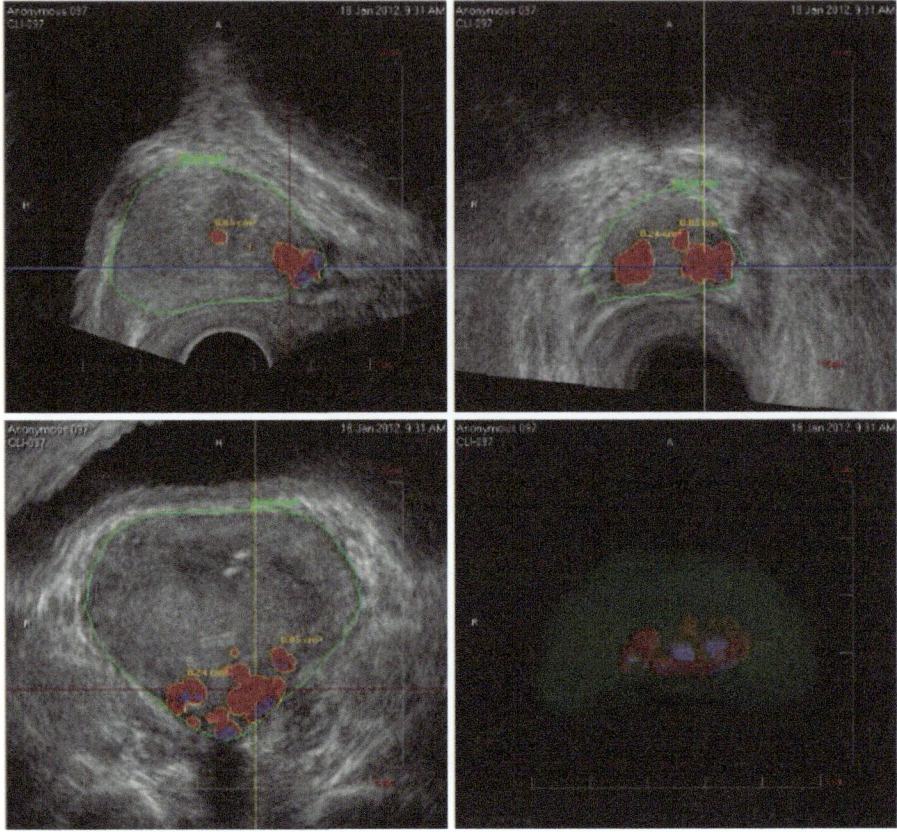

Fig. 5.3 3D visualization of suspicious areas, *highlighted in red or purple*, following HistoScanning analysis

5.4 Perineal HistoScanning Targeted Biopsy

The perineal HistoScanning-guided biopsy is performed with the patient in a dorsal lithotomy position under general or spinal anesthesia. A brachytherapy template grid fixed to a cradle is placed next to the perineum and used as a guide. Using the information from the HS projection reports, the biopsy needle is directed under direct guidance by a triplane ultrasound probe (BK 8848 probe, Analogic Corp, Peabody MA, USA). Depending on local practice, template-guided systematic Bx, template-guided HS targeted, as well as extended mapping biopsies can be performed without auxiliary procedures.

In comparison to the transrectal approach, the perineal biopsy technique might reduce variables that can influence the needle placement. Furthermore, longitudinal biopsy punches following the axis of the prostate seem to allow more accurate sampling of the anterior part.

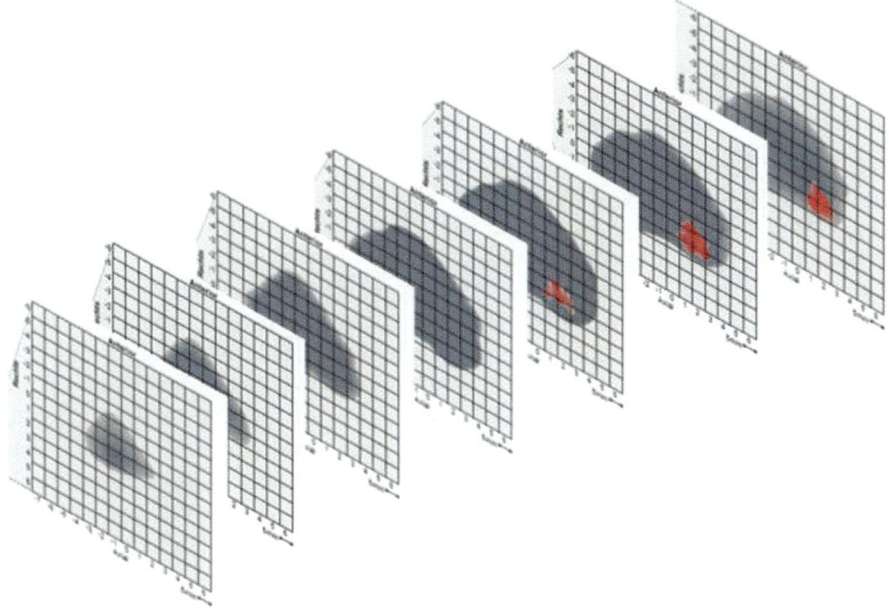

Fig. 5.4 HistoScanning reconstructs a quasi-3D volumetric grid (transversal slice report) with suspicious areas *highlighted*. Based on these HistoScanning images, the metrical report (0.2 mm resolution) allows stereotactical guidance of perineal prostate biopsy procedures

5.5 Current Evidence

Although multiple studies have shown the promise of adding HistoScanning to a targeted biopsy program, the value of HS is still under debate. Recent publications report controversial outcome of HS in routine clinical practice. De Coninck et al. reported findings in 41/94 men who underwent a transrectal prostate biopsy supplemented with cognitive-targeted biopsies in suspicious regions based on prostate HS. The authors found that in men with prostate cancer, HistoScanning-based biopsy was 4.5 times more likely to detect cancer than systematic biopsy ($p < 0.0001$). Logistic regression analysis determined that the HistoScanning lesion volume was the most significant predictor for positive biopsy outcomes with an odds ratio of 2.9 ($p = 0.022$) for every 1 ml increase. These results seem to be contrary to recent data on 198 men who received a nontargeted transrectal prostate biopsy. The retrospective correlation of histopathologic findings with HistoScanning analysis in this cohort revealed only a low predictive accuracy (AUC 0.58) of HistoScanning [11]. But large discrepancy between the volume of prostate sextants and the corresponding HS volume might account for a relevant sampling error. The nontargeted setting of the transrectal biopsy rather confounds evaluation of HS results because cancer detection is determined by the systematic approach, not by HS analysis. This underlines the necessity of detailed biopsy planning and favors alternative modalities such as perineal (targeted) biopsies. In this regard, Javed et al. report on the diagnostic characteristics of HS in 57 patients who underwent transperineal template biopsy. Again, according to sextant analysis, no relationship was demonstrated between targeted biopsies of HS positive regions and the tumor burden within the corresponding sextant assessed [8]. Controversially, in 80 men ($n = 28$ with prostate cancer) who underwent a systematic 14-core transrectal biopsy supplemented with a targeted transperineal biopsy (maximum nine cores per three locations), the targeted biopsy detected 82 % of all cancers, similar to the detection rate of the 14-core systematic biopsy [6]. Further data on targeted repeat biopsies in 97 patients showed on prostate sector level sensitivity, specificity, predictive accuracy, negative, and positive predictive values of 44, 83, 80, 95, and 17 %, respectively (Hamann MF, et al. 2014). Additionally at patient level, histopathologic analysis detects prostatitis, HG-PIN, and ASAP in 73, 18, and 5 %, respectively. But again, analysis of HS suspicious volume in this series showed no significant impact on BX outcome. Finally, these results are supported by a small study that compared the tumor volumes estimated by HS with that measured in corresponding prostatectomy specimen [8]. In contrast to the results from initial as well as recent validation of HS in radical prostatectomy studies [12, 9], the authors concluded that HS fails to identify prostate cancer accurately in the clinical setting.

In conclusion, HS signals allow qualitative rather than quantitative interpretation when transferred to biopsy planning. With respect to the high NPV throughout all prostate sectors, data might suggest to spare biopsies in non-HS-positive regions. Corresponding PB scheme would theoretically achieve appropriate sampling rather by increasing core numbers than by targeting proper geographical locations, because a common 12-core biopsy potentially detects the majority of clinically significant cancers with 80 % sensitivity, as shown in a step-section analysis of 164 autopsies [5]. In this study, the authors concluded that the ability to detect cancer was related more to the sampling location (peripheral, lateral, and apical cores) than to the number of biopsy cores taken. Those results clearly underline the benefit of HistoScanning providing an objective ultrasound meta-analysis detecting prostate regions that harbor abnormal tissues. But a sophisticated biopsy technique is needed to harvest the gains of the HistoScanning.

5.6   Summary

HistoScanning is an ultrasound-based tissue characterization application that uses 3D raw RF data from a clinical TRUS examination to visualize and locate tissues suspected of harboring prostate cancer. HistoScanning analysis uses ultrasound backscatter properties and statistical classifiers that were trained from detailed pathology to identify the presence of prostate cancer and other suspicious tissues. These tools, which are connected to standard ultrasound equipment, hold the promise of detecting the lesions of clinical significance irrespective of observer quality. Sophisticated biopsy planning based on HistoScanning results might reduce patient burden of a systematic biopsy procedure while still detecting the majority of clinically significant cancers. Future trials must focus on the comparison of HistoScanning to standard of care biopsy procedures to further demonstrate the value of using ultrasound-based tissue characterization as a tool to improve prostate biopsies.

References

1. Aigner F, Schafer G, Steiner E, et al. Value of enhanced transrectal ultrasound targeted biopsy for prostate cancer diagnosis: a retrospective data analysis. World J Urol. 2012;30:341–6.
2. Braeckman J, Autier P, Garbar C, et al. Computer-aided ultrasonography (HistoScanning): a novel technology for locating and characterizing prostate cancer. BJU Int. 2008;101:293–8.
3. Braeckman J, Autier P, Soviany C, et al. The accuracy of transrectal ultrasonography supplemented with computer-aided ultrasonography for detecting small prostate cancers. BJU Int. 2008;102:1560–5.
4. Grabski B, Baeurle L, Loch A, Wefer B, Paul U, Loch T. Computerized transrectal ultrasound of the prostate in a multicenter setup (C-TRUS-MS): detection of cancer after multiple negative systematic random and in primary biopsies. World J Urol. 2011;29(5):573–9.
5. Haas GP, Delongchamps NB, Jones RF, Chandan V, Serio AM, Vickers AJ, Jumbelic M, Threatte G, Korets R, Lilja H, de la Roza G. Needle biopsies on autopsy prostates: sensitivity of cancer detection based on true prevalence. J Natl Cancer Inst. 2007;99(19):1484–9.
6. Hamann MF, Hamann C, Schenk E, et al. Computer-aided (HistoScanning) biopsies versus conventional transrectal ultrasound guided prostate biopsies: do targeted biopsy schemes improve the cancer detection rate? Urology. 2013;81:370–5.
7. Heijmink S, van Moerkerk H, Kiemeney L, et al. A comparison of the diagnostic performance of systematic versus ultrasound-guided biopsies of prostate cancer. Eur Radiol. 2006; 16(4):927–38.
8. Javed S, Chadwick E, Edwards AA, Beveridge S, Laing R, Bott S, Eden C, Langley S. Does prostate HistoScanning™ play a role in detecting prostate cancer in routine clinical practice? Results from three independent studies. BJU Int. 2014;114(4):541–8. doi:10.1111/bju.12568.
9. Macek P, Barret E, Sanchez-Salas R, Galiano M, Rozet F, Ahallal Y, Gaya JM, Durant M, Mascle L, Giedelman C, Lunelli L, Validire P, Nesvadba M, Cathelineau X. Prostate histoscanning in clinically localized biopsy proven prostate cancer: an accuracy study. J Endourol. 2014;28(3):371–6.
10. Salomon G, Schiffmann J. Real-time elastography for the detection of prostate cancer. Curr Urol Rep. 2014;15(3):392.
11. Schiffmann J, Tennstedt P, Fischer J, Tian Z, Beyer B, Boehm K, Sun M, Gandaglia G, Michl U, Graefen M, Salomon G. Does HistoScanning™ predict positive results in prostate biopsy? A retrospective analysis of 1,188 sextants of the prostate. World J Urol. 2014;32(4):925–30.
12. Simmons LA, Autier P, Zát'ura F, Braeckman J, Peltier A, Romic I, Stenzl A, Treurnicht K, Walker T, Nir D, Moore CM, Emberton M. Detection, localisation and characterisation of prostate cancer by prostate HistoScanning(™). BJU Int. 2012;110(1):28–35.

Noninvasive Radio Frequency for Early Diagnosis of Prostate Cancer

6

Carlo Bellorofonte, Claudio Cesana, and Luciano Morselli

Contents

6.1 Introduction

Prostate cancer is the second most prevalent cancer in the adult male and the sixth most common cause of cancer death [1]. Prevalence of the disease is considered to increase over the years. In 2015, the American Cancer Society estimate 220,800 new prostate cancer cases, of which 27,250 will be death cases. One man over seven will be diagnosed with prostate cancer during his lifetime. Early diagnosis of prostate cancer is a highly debated issue, and screening is not considered worthwhile

C. Bellorofonte (✉) • C. Cesana
Department of Urology, Columbus Clinic, Milan, Italy
e-mail: bellorof@gmail.com

L. Morselli
Kimea Pte. Ltd., Singapore, Singapore

© Springer International Publishing Switzerland 2015
S. Thüroff, C.G. Chaussy (eds.), *Focal Therapy of Prostate Cancer:
An Emerging Strategy for Minimally Invasive, Staged Treatment*,
DOI 10.1007/978-3-319-14160-2_6

because of the unfavorable number of patients that need to be diagnosed and treated to save every one. Any how, prostate cancer diagnosis remains a very important issue because of the different screening programs that are adopted in the most developed countries.

Prostate-specific antigen (PSA) testing has been instrumental to increase the diagnosis of an organ-confined disease amenable to cure. Notwithstanding the recent development of novel treatment regimens, metastatic disease still remains incurable, and all the related treatments are actually palliative. PSA test is currently used in a way to offer high sensitivity and low specificity; consequently more than half of patients undergoing biopsy are found negative.

PCA3 testing has been proposed as an adjunct to PSA for early diagnosis of prostate cancer for its larger discriminatory power, although it needs prostatic massage and the high costs have limited its widespread adoption [2]. Still today, only in 17 % of patients prostate cancer is suspected after a digital rectal examination.

Diagnostic tests for prostate cancer are not only used for early diagnosis but are frequently used in follow-up of prostate cancer treatments such as radical prostatectomy, radiotherapy, hormonal treatment, and chemotherapy.

Research on the physical properties of cancerous tissues helped identify a number of parameters characteristic of neoplastic tissues that could possibly be used for diagnostic purposes. The relatively poor background of the medical community in fundamental physics should not underscore the importance of this research area. We just have to consider that all imaging techniques (ultrasonography, CT scan, MRI) that we currently use in our patients are based on the different physical properties of cancerous tissue.

A number of research laboratories are actively working on the development of diagnostic technology based on the use of low-energy electromagnetic radiation. This is a relatively novel approach that aims at identifying the presence of cancerous lesions without necessarily providing imaging of the observed tumor.

From the electromagnetic (EM) point of view, tumors have higher water content than normal surrounding cells due to cellular necrosis, increased and irregular vascularization, and alteration of nutrients. The EM evidence is in the electrical conductivity and permittivity of many tumors with respect to the normal surrounding tissues; this contrast is further enhanced by the size and development stage of the tumor. Investigations on the EM properties of tumor tissues have been of interest for over a century with several evidences on the feasibility of the usage of EM as diagnostic tool. In spite of the usage of microwaves (>1 GHz) for imaging in place of (or complementary to) conventional CT or MRI imaging diagnostics, there has been some early research on the usage of devices within the frequency range 300–500 MHz where tissue absorption peaks due to water and sodium content of malignant tissues.

In this context, TRIMprob was the first diagnostic device made available in Italy over a decade ago for routine usage in clinics. Accuracy appeared to exceed 50 % in both sensitivity and specificity; its negative predictive value raised the interests for its potential usage in the reduction of the number of unnecessary biopsies [3–5]. TRIMprob was still an investigational device, but it shed light on the diagnostic capability by coupling a probe with tumor tissues.

ESO-MED 8G is a new-generation diagnostic device for the extracorporeal diagnosis of prostate cancer that was developed in Italy and introduced in the market in 2012. Based on the same concept of coupling tissues with a probe maneuvered by the clinician, ESO-MED 8G is largely improved in usage and reliability, with high diagnostic accuracy reaching sensitivity and specificity levels above 95 %.

In this chapter, after recalling the TRIMprob studies made on prostate cancer in 2005, 2007, and 2008, a new clinical study is presented, done with the objective to evaluate ESO-MED 8G diagnostic accuracy.

6.2   EM Diagnostics: A Review

The knowledge of the electrical property of tissues has been of interest for over a century. Measurements and models have been developed to account for behaviors of biological tissues either normal or pathological [6–9]. Microscopic description of the electrical properties of cells is complicated by the variety and the distribution of cell type and organs' shape; therefore, a macroscopic approach is most often adopted to establish the specific conductivity and relative permittivity of biological systems. At macroscopic level, these properties are further complicated by several factors such as tissue orientation, frequency, inhomogeneity, and physiological factors. Cole-Cole model that accounts for relaxation time has been validated in different settings and for various tissues. The model can extrapolate the macroscopic properties at high frequency [7, 8], and EM parameters have been evaluated and validated in great details for breast carcinoma [10].

Imaging methods based on non-ionizing EM waves have been investigated over the last decades, mostly for breast cancer as the local geometry is somewhat simpler than the remaining part of the body. Normal breast tissues are translucent to microwaves (as mostly low-water content fat tissue); the high dielectric contrast of malignant tissues compared to the surrounding area (at least 5:1) makes breast tumor an excellent disease for optimizing microwave modeling and imaging [11].

Active microwave (>1 GHz) imaging techniques for tumors are based on two main methods: tomography and radar-like. The goal of tomography is to recover the dielectric property of the breast from multiple views using narrowband signals [11]. Ultrawideband (UWB) radar seeks to identify the presence and the location of any meaningful scatterer in the breast [12], and similar to tomography, multiple views can be used to image these anomalous scatterers to let the clinician have a diagnostic tool that can be easily integrated with the preexisting imaging devices [13]. Numerical modeling for heterogeneous (up to 20 % heterogeneity) and realistic propagating medium proved that shallow (3–4 cm depth) and small (below 0.5 cm) tumors can be detected by UWB radar system over 4–8 GHz bandwidth [12]. Since all these EM methods aim to provide an image of inner body for diagnostic, the main drawbacks are the cost for equipment/acquisition that is comparable with diagnostic imaging tools routinely employed (e.g., CT, MRI, PET).

In the range of frequency around 500 MHz, there is a peak of absorption, around 300–500 MHz, namely, due to the increase of water and sodium in malignant tissues (see, e.g., [6] or [8]). In hyperthermia [14], the anomaly around this frequency range is used to locally raise the temperature in order to induce cytotoxic effects and make malignant cells more vulnerable to ionizing radiation and chemical toxins as adjuvant to radiotherapy and/or chemotherapy [15]. The diagnostic use of EM in the frequency range around 434 MHz is for thermoacoustic tomography [16]. Once again, the dielectric properties of tissues in this frequency range make the EM radiation to be absorbed differently of healthy/tumor tissues. When radiated, the tissue expansion produces pressure waves that are measured at surface and are used in thermoacoustic tomography to image the biologic tissues on the basis of its different absorption of EM radiation for healthy or tumor tissues.

Even if the prostate is fairly complex for EM imaging as the tissues are much more complex and heterogeneous compared to the breast, it has the advantage of being geometrically uniquely located regardless of the patient's height and weight. This property favors EM methods around 500 MHz as the EM field couples with prostate and provides altered response when in presence of tumor tissues. Even if narrowband signals below 500 MHz are not suited for imaging due to the lack of resolution, malignant tissues have large electrical contrasts compared to the surrounding tissues such that these can closely couple with a radiating antenna provided that tumors are shallow enough (say, below 5 cm if permittivity ranges within 5–10 as for fat tissues) as for prostate or early-stage tumors in breast [12]. Alteration in antenna's coupling in prostate cancer detection can be diagnostic of pathological tissues provided that this coupling can be measured and related to tissues properties. This is the frequency range considered herein with encouraging clinical results.

6.3 History

History of technology begins with an equipment called TRIMprob. TRIMprob is a diagnostic equipment composed of an oscillator embedded in a cylindrical probe that couples with tissues and a spectrum analyzer paired with dedicated software for the analysis of the frequency and power of probe oscillator.

The TRIMprob generates harmonic waves with three frequency components (465, 930, and 1,395 MHz), and it is moved over the perineum. After preliminary clinical trials that allowed to determine the prostate diagnosis method, in 2005 Bellorofonte published the first seminal paper on the clinical outcomes from the usage of EM diagnosis for prostate cancer [3]. The interaction between the EM field emitted by the probe and cancerous tissue results in a decrease of the signal intensity at 465 MHz (Fig. 6.1, Table 6.1), whereas the signal at 930 and 1,395 remains almost unchanged.

Power is measured in arbitrary units ranging between 255 and 0. Mean values and standard deviation data are presented. Analysis of the patient groups shows significant differences at 465 and 930 MHz, while no significant difference was seen at 1,395 MHz.

Preliminary evaluation of TRIMprob accuracy showed a sensitivity of 95.5 % and a specificity of 42.7 %, with a positive predictive value (PPV) of 63.6 % and a negative predictive value (NPV) of 89.8 % (Table 6.2) [3].

465 MHZ

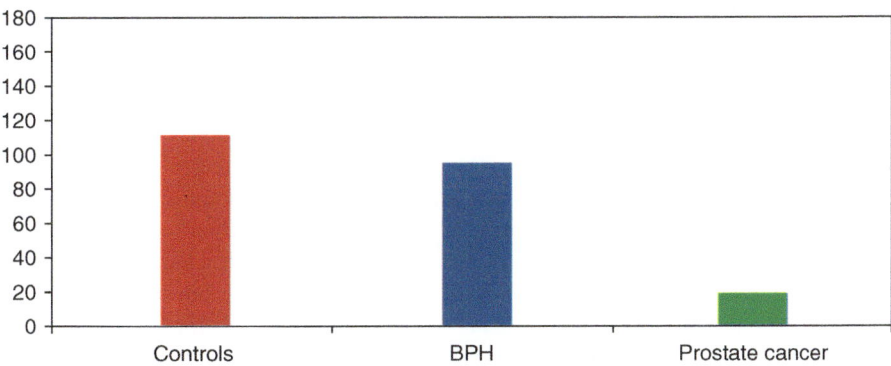

Fig. 6.1 TRIMprob signal amplitude (mean values and standard deviation) at 465 MHz in control patients with BPH and PSA <4.0 ng/ml and patients with a biopsy-proven diagnosis of prostate cancer

Table 6.1   Field level measured by the TRIMprob at 465, 930, and 1,395 MHz

	No. of patients (757)	Prostate cancer on biopsy	Average (SD)		
			465 MHz	930 MHz	1,395 MHz
Controls	163	n.a.	110.7 (36.4)	45.1 (18.2)	49.7 (16.3)
BPH with PSA ≤4.0 ng/ml and normal DRE	228	n.a.	94.0 (45.9)	41.8 (19.4)	48.5 (13.8)
BPH with PSA >4.0 ng/ml and normal DRE	167	31	51.8 (51.9)	37.2 (21.4)	50.7 (16.7)
Abnormal DRE	91	77	10.5 (19.7)	36.2 (18.4)	48.9 (12.5)
Prostate cancer	108	n.a.	19.2 (29.7)	36.0 (19.1)	52.2 (14.7)
One-way ANOVA			$p \le 0.0001$	$p \le 0.0001$	$p \le 0.247$

Table 6.2   Sensitivity, specificity, and positive and negative predictive value of individual diagnostic parameters

	Sensitivity (%)	Specificity (%)	PPV (%)	NPV (%)
TRIMprob (cut off a 50)	95.4	42.7	63.6	89.8
PSA (≥4.0 ng/ml)	94.4	7.3	47.2	60.0
PSA ratio (18 %)	80.4	46.2	59.4	70.6
DRE	68.9	80.2	76.0	73.8
TRUS	84.3	52.6	62.3	78.2

From Ref. [3]

In 2007 Da Pozzo L. et al. evaluated the accuracy of the TRIMprob in a multicenter prospective study. The authors concluded that TRIMprob increases the accuracy of PSA or DRE results, and with its high NPV, it might be useful to reduce the indications for prostatic biopsy or repeated series of biopsies in patients suspected of having prostate cancer (Table 6.3) [4].

In 2008 Tubaro et al. evaluated the accuracy of the TRIMprob test, total PSA, free/total PSA ratio, DRE, and transrectal ultrasonography (TRUS) in the diagnosis of prostate neoplasm in a prospective study, confirming the data previously published by Bellorofonte in Table 6.4.

The diagnostic accuracy of the TRIMprob device was tested in the diagnosis of other tumors including bladder, colon, and breast cancer although most of the published data refer to prostate cancer. The published results clearly demonstrated a good diagnostic accuracy with an interesting balance between sensitivity and specificity. The cons of TRIMprob consisted in its long learning curve; this made its adoption quite difficult. The industrial story behind the TRIMprob is beyond the scope of this chapter; although the device failed from a commercial standpoint, the science behind it is, in our opinion, here to stay.

Table 6.3 The sensitivity specificity, PPV, NPV, and accuracy of TRIMprob, DRE, and %fPSA in 188 patients

Test	Sensitivity	Specificity	PPV	NPV	Accuracy
TRIMprob	80	51	44	84	60
DRE	41	89	64	75	73
%fPSA (threshold 18)	79	46	79	46	58
TRIMprob + DRE	92	47	46	92	61

From Ref. [4]

Table 6.4 Sensitivity, specificity, positive and negative predictive value, and accuracy of individual and associated diagnostic parameters

Parameter	Sensitivity	Specificity	Positive predictive value	Negative predictive value	Accuracy
Individual parameters					
TRIMprob	0.86	0.63	0.60	0.88	0.72
Total PSA (≥4.0 ng/mL)	0.90	0.16	0.41	0.73	0.45
Free/total PSA (≤0.18)	0.78	0.34	0.35	0.72	0.50
DRE	0.40	0.88	0.69	0.69	0.69
TRUS	0.36	0.79	0.69	0.48	0.55
Coin toss	0.45	0.54	0.36	0.63	0.55
Associated parameters					
TRIMprob + DRE	0.96	0.57	0.59	0.95	0.72
Total PSA + DRE	0.96	0.13	0.42	0.82	0.46
Free/total PSA + DRE	0.81	0.53	0.51	0.82	0.64

From Ref. [5]

PSA prostate-specific antigen, *DRE* digital rectal examination, *TRUS* transrectal ultrasound

6.4   ESO-MED 8G

ESO-MED 8G in Fig. 6.2 is an electro medical device, designed and manufactured by MEDIELMA, Italy, for the electromagnetic diagnosis of cancer. Even if it is conceptually different from TRIMprob, the maneuvering of the probe of ESO-MED 8G system is similar to TRIMprob. ESO-MED 8G is less sensitive to environmental noise, more reliable, and less operator dependent. This makes the ESO-MED 8G a good candidate as a diagnostic device for the early diagnosis of prostate cancer.

Herein we present the first exploratory analysis of the ESO-MED 8G diagnostic accuracy in patients at risk of prostate cancer by using the same experimental setting as for TRIMprob.

The device is composed of one transmitting probe, a receiver apparatus, and a diagnostic station with a proprietary processing software. The probe is a portable device powered by internal batteries able to generate a low-power radiofrequency

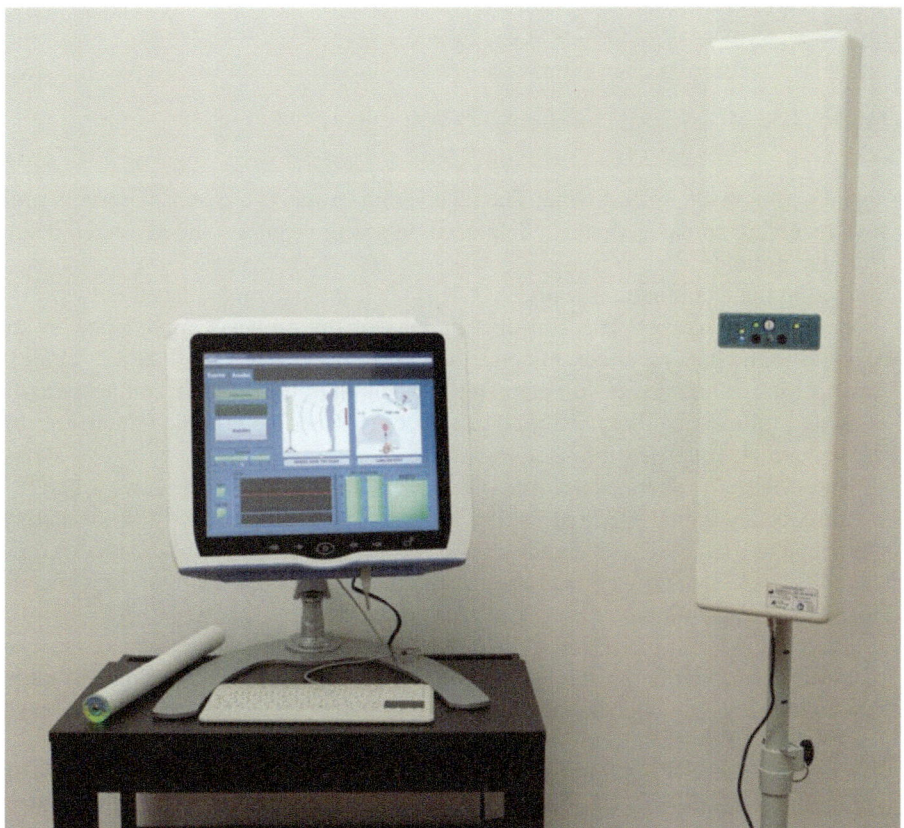

Fig. 6.2 ESO-MED 8G components (*left* to *right*): probe, diagnostic station, receiver

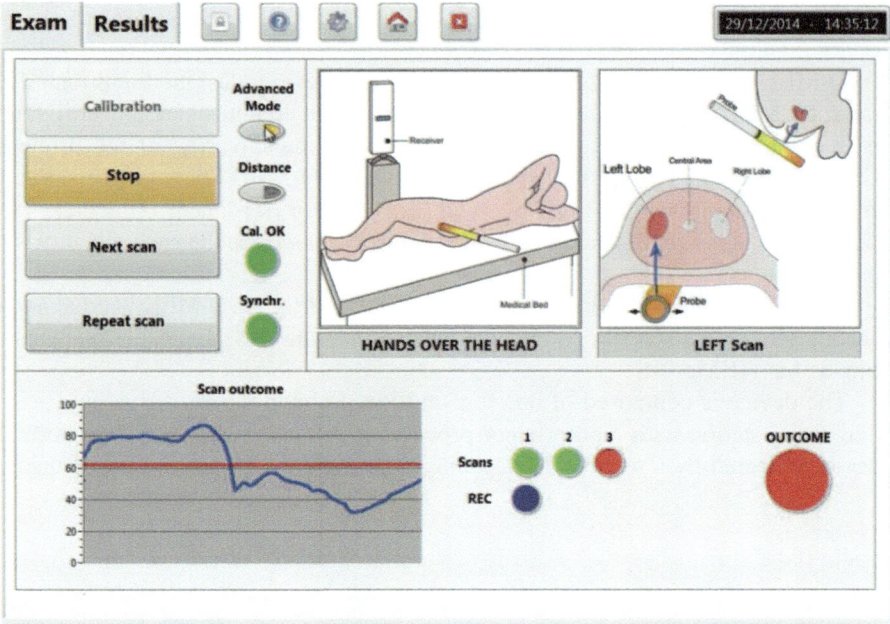

Fig. 6.3 ESO-MED 8G diagnostic station screen showing a positive exam

signal within medical ISM band. The receiver apparatus is a base station with multiple receiving antennas that can be placed on a wall or on a stand at a fixed height from the ground.

During the examinations with ESO-MED 8G, the patient is placed between the probe and the receiver. The emitting antenna of the probe is approached by the operator to the patient's body in correspondence of the anatomical area of interest. The operator adjusts the position and the inclination of the probe in contact with the body and follows the diagnostic indications of the specific graphical interface that guide the probe maneuvering (see Fig. 6.3).

ESO-MED 8G operates according to the principles described above where the radiofrequency signal radiated by the probe is coupled differently with healthy/pathological tissues. The different level of coupling is detected by the receiver and then processed by software that allows a graphical representation through specific diagnostic indicators.

The clinical examination is noninvasive and well tolerated as being extracorporeal. Moreover the diagnostic test is not harmful as it uses non-ionizing EM radiations with very low intensity, frequency in 423–443 MHz ISM range, and power level below the one of a cellular phone.

The outcome of the diagnostic tests is displayed automatically by the ESO-MED 8G. It compares the values of power received by several receiving antennas with a predetermined threshold. In particular, the software provides the following outcomes:

- Negative examination: the power received by antennas is never below the threshold for the duration of the examination.
- Suspected cancer: the power received by antennas is below the threshold for a relevant time interval. The ESO-MED 8G system provides the user with an automatic interpretation of the exam.

Three scans are saved for each patient in correspondence of the prostate anatomical parts (right lobe, left lobe, and central adenoma).

6.5 ESO-MED 8G Clinical Study

ESO-MED clinical data for the diagnosis of prostate cancer were collected at the department of urology of the Columbus Clinic in Milan, Italy, from November 2012 to November 2013 on 624 patients. The group of patients examined was composed of 502 healthy patients (control group) and 122 patients with histologically proven prostate cancer (clinical group). The examination performed with ESO-MED 8G did not lead to any adverse event. The examination procedure was always easily performed, with an overall duration of between 5 and 10 min and without any patient discomfort.

Sensitivity, specificity, accuracy, positive predictive value (PPV), and negative predictive value (NPV) were calculated from the clinical trials. The results obtained were then compared with those reported in literature relating to other most commonly used diagnostic tests for prostate cancer (PSA, digital rectal examination, and transrectal ultrasound).

Simple descriptive statistics (mean value and standard deviation) for the signal values measured during the survey period were obtained for two groups of patients analyzed: control and clinical groups. Mean value and standard deviation were calculated for each healthy patient and compared with the values calculated for each deseased patient.

Finally, the ROC curve (receiver operating characteristic) for the variable described earlier has been obtained in a nonparametric way, and the area under the curve (AUC-ROC) has been calculated. More specifically, AUC-ROC can vary from 0.5 to 1, and the values assumed denote a good discrimination as more as they are close to 1, while values close to 0.5 identify the test as unreliable.

The mean age and standard deviation of the subject considered in this study are 42.2 ± 26.8 years. The group of cases consisted of patients with confirmed histologic diagnosis of prostate cancer. Gleason grades were stratified as follows:

- 60 cases of prostate cancer Gleason 6 $(3+3)$
- 42 cases of prostate cancer Gleason 7 $(3+4)$
- 14 cases of prostate cancer Gleason 7 $(4+3)$
- 3 cases of prostate cancer Gleason 8 $(4+4)$
- 3 cases of prostate cancer Gleason 9 $(4+5)$

Table 6.5 Minimum power values of the signal measured with ESO-MED 8G at the frequency of 433 MHz

	N° considered tracks	Mean value [dBm]	Standard dev. [dB]
Healthy patient	1,506	−29.4	5.0
Patient with cancer	366	−56.8	4.7

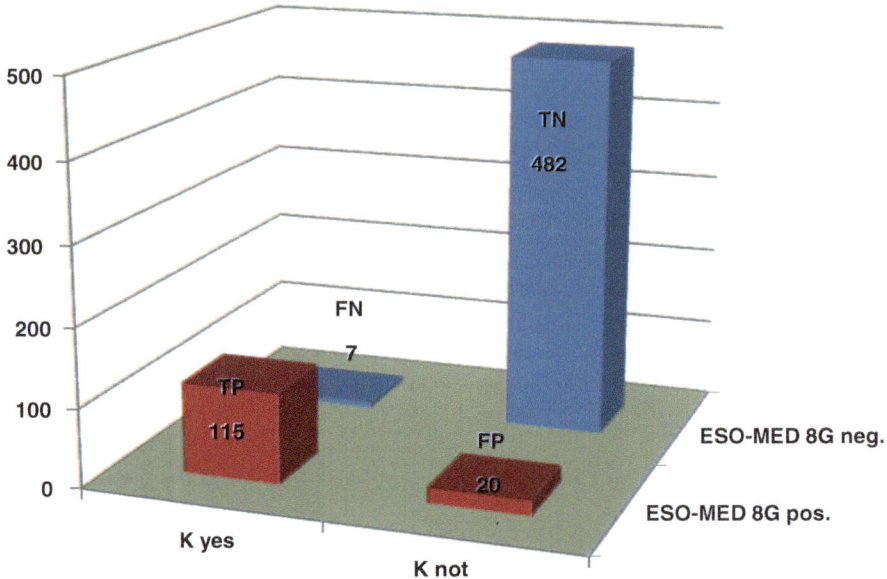

Fig. 6.4 Diagnostic outcomes on prostate obtained with the ESO-MED 8G device

The analysis of all scans recorded (3 for each patient for a total of 1,872 scans) revealed a significant difference in the value of the signal at a frequency of 433 MHz between healthy patients and those affected by prostate cancer (Table 6.5).

Analysis of the results of the ESO-MED 8G diagnosis showed 489 (78.4 %) negative results (TN + FN), where 482 out of 489 were from the control group. 135 exams (21.6 %) proved to be positive, of which 115 (TP) patients have histologically proven prostate cancer. Figure 6.4 shows the statistical distribution of the ESO-MED diagnostic results. Of note are the significantly low number of false positive (FP) and false negative (FN).

The analysis of clinical outcomes obtained with the ESO-MED 8G diagnostic device provides a sensitivity of 94.3 % and a specificity of 96.0 %. The accuracy of the system is 95.7 %, while the positive and negative predictive values are 85.2 and 98.6 %, respectively. Table 6.6 summarizes the results obtained compared with those of the most common tests used for the diagnosis of prostate cancer: PSA, digital rectal examination (DRE), and transrectal ultrasound (TRUS).

Table 6.6 Sensitivity, specificity, positive and negative predictive value, and accuracy for ESO-MED 8G, PSA, DRE and TRUS

	Sensitivity	Specificity	PPV	NPV	Accuracy
ESO-MED 8G	0.94	0.96	0.85	0.98	0.96
PSA	0.90	0.16	0.41	0.73	0.45
DRE	0.40	0.88	0.69	0.69	0.69
TRUS	0.36	0.79	0.69	0.48	0.55

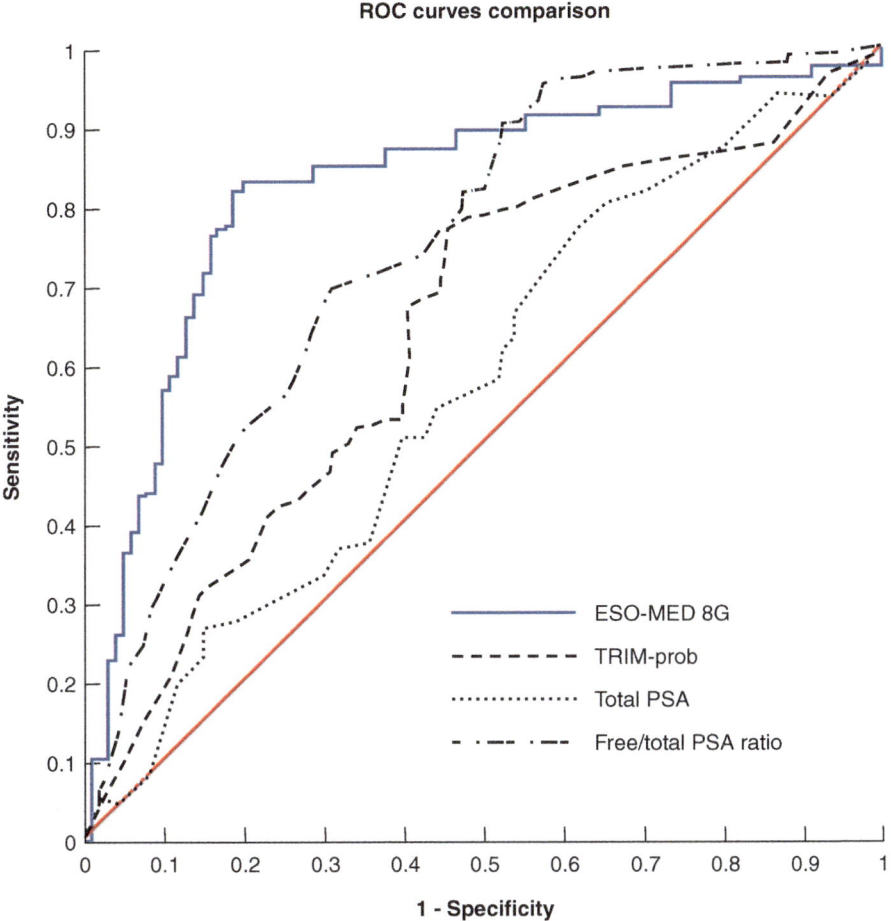

Fig. 6.5 Receiver operating characteristic (ROC) curve of ESO-MED 8G in comparison with other tests (TRIMprob, total PSA, and free/total PSA ratio, all obtained from Ref. [3])

The ROC curve is in Fig. 6.5 with a value of AUC-ROC for ESO-MED 8G equal to 0.92. The same figure compares the ROC curves of TRIMprob (at 465 MHz), total PSA, and free/total PSA ratio extracted from Ref. [3]. Even if the results are from two different clinical trials, Fig. 6.5 confirms the remarkable benefits of the ESO-MED 8G technology.

The main purpose of this exploratory study was to determine the ESO-MED 8G performance in a non-blind setting. Different from TRIMprob where the diagnostic interpretations from three frequencies are left to the skill of the operators, the new ESO-MED 8G device performs an automated evaluation that, to some extent, cannot be influenced by the investigator.

A remarkable difference in attenuation (approx. 20–25 dB) of the signal between the healthy subjects (mean value, −29.4 dBm) and the patients affected by prostate cancer (mean value, −56.8 dBm) was observed by analyzing the signal levels measured by the ESO-MED 8G. This signal strength difference is significant from a physical standpoint, and it suggests that the EM diagnostic setup is able to distinguish healthy from pathological tissues within the frequency range of good EM penetration capability in tissues. In this clinical study, an optimal threshold value has been identified, giving the best trade off in terms of sensitivity and specificity.

With this optimized threshold value, the diagnostic performance of the ESO-MED 8G was interesting from a clinical standpoint. In particular, a very high negative predictive value (NPV = 98 %) was found that can be attributed to a high capability of the device in detecting the healthy subjects. This is a very important characteristic because it justifies the use of ESO-MED 8G as a first screening tool able to detect with high probability the healthy subjects. In case of negative results, ESO-MED 8G avoids patients to incur in further examination that can be time-consuming, invasive, and uncomfortable. On the other hand, if the examination was positive, this should be interpreted as an alarm of a possible presence of cancer and this supports the suggestion for the patient to execute more in-depth examination (e.g., biopsy).

6.6   ESO-Prost 8G: A Further Step Ahead

Subsequent to the aforementioned 1-year study (November 2012 to November 2013) using ESO-MED 8G, the ESO-Prost 8G was introduced in the market by MEDIELMA.

ESO-Prost is the system presently used in the urology department of Columbus Clinic (Milan, Italy) (Figs. 6.6 and 6.7).

This new system is part of the ESO-MED 8G family, and it is dedicated and optimized to the prostate examination. ESO-Prost 8G includes all the features of the ESO-MED 8G with many enhancement that makes it even easier to use.

The main advantages of ESO-Prost compared to the multiorgan ESO-MED are:

- Much less room space required
- Simpler probe maneuvering
- Better graphical user interface dedicated to prostate examination

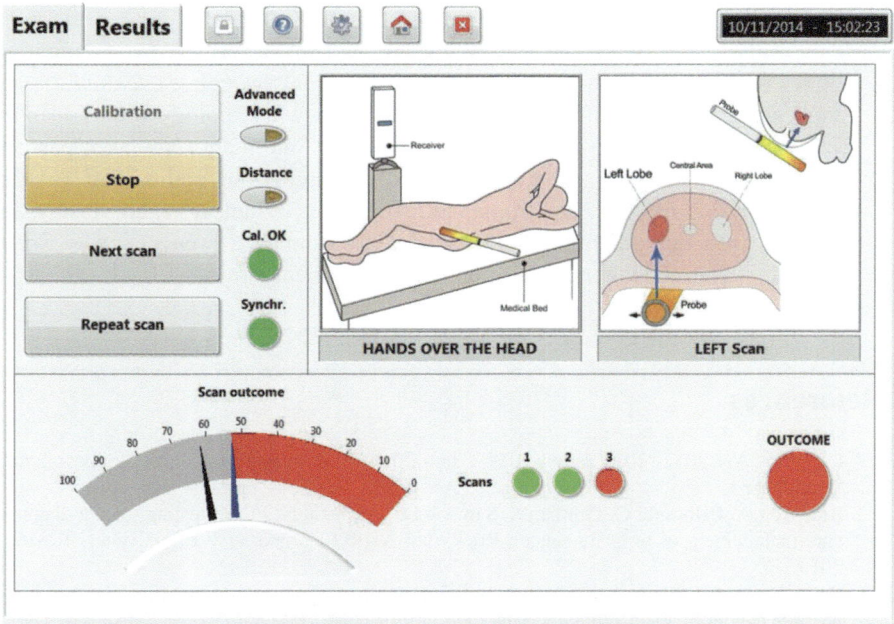

Fig. 6.6 ESO-Prost 8G diagnostic station screen showing a positive exam

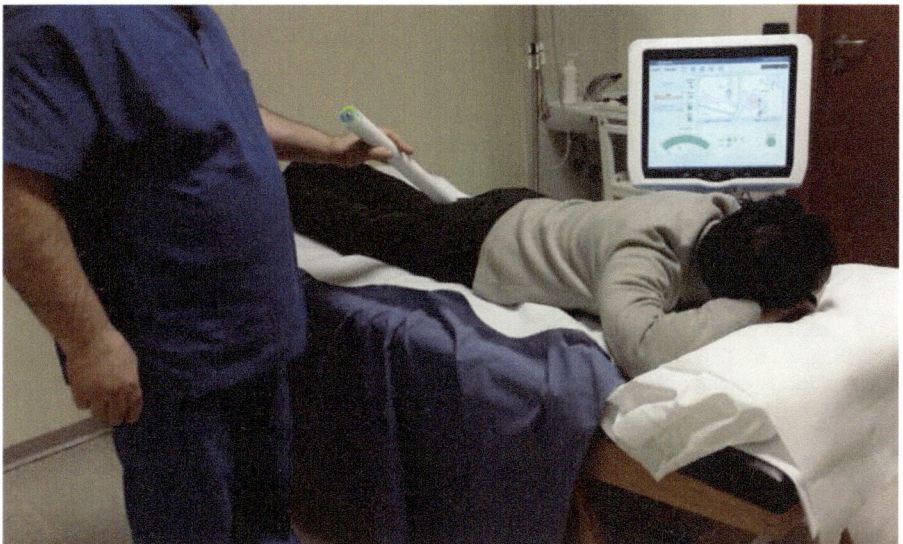

Fig. 6.7 Example of ESO-Prost 8G exam

Conclusions

This is the dawn of new era in which applied physics entered our outpatient clinics from a totally new perspective. Any real breakthrough is a teamwork, and it takes much longer time than anticipated. This new technology would open the road toward new diagnostic devices, possibly fully automatic. However, past and current clinical outcomes are undoubtedly helping the enthusiasm for this early-diagnosis method. Electromagnetic diagnosis of cancer is here to stay, and research into this scientific field remains a fascinating area that was finally translated from the laboratory bench to the outpatient clinic.

References

1. GLOBOCAN 2012, 2014 [cited 2014 2 Feb 2014]. Available from: http://globocan.iarc.fr/Default.aspx.
2. Bradley LA, Palomaki G, Gutman S, Samson DJ, Aronson N. PCA3 testing for the diagnosis and management of prostate cancer. Rockville: AHRQ Comparative Effectiveness Reviews; 2013.
3. Bellorofonte C, Vedruccio C, Tombolini P, Ruoppolo M, Tubaro A. Non-invasive detection of prostate cancer by electromagnetic interaction. Eur Urol. 2005;47(1):29–37; discussion 37.
4. Da Pozzo L, Scattoni V, Mazzoccoli B, Rigatti P, Manferrari F, Martorana G, et al. Tissue-resonance interaction method for the noninvasive diagnosis of prostate cancer: analysis of a multicentre clinical evaluation. BJU Int. 2007;100(5):1055–9.
5. Tubaro A, De Nunzio C, Trucchi A, Stoppacciaro A, Miano L. The electromagnetic detection of prostatic cancer: evaluation of diagnostic accuracy. Urology. 2008;72(2):340–4.
6. Foster KRS, Schwan HP. Dielectric properties of tissues. In: Handbook of biological effects of electromagnetic field. New York: CRC Press; 1996.
7. Gabriel SL, Lau RW, Gabriel C. The dielectric properties of biological tissues: III. Parametric models for the dielectric spectrum of tissues. Phys Med Biol. 1996;41(11):2271–93.
8. Foster KRS, Schwan HP. Dielectric properties of tissues and biological materials: a critical review. Crit Rev Biomed Eng. 1989;17:25–104.
9. Vaupel PK, Kallinowski F, Okunieff P. Blood flow, oxygen and nutrient supply, and metabolic microenvironment of human tumors: a review. Cancer Res. 1989;40:6449–65.
10. Surowiec AJ, Stuchly SS, Barr JB, Swarup A. Dielectric properties of breast carcinoma and the surrounding tissues. IEEE Trans Biomed Eng. 1988;35(4):257–63.
11. Fear EC, Hagness SC, Meaney PM, Okoniewski M, Stuchly MA. Enhancing breast tumor detection with near field imaging. IEEE Microwave Mag. 2002;3:8–56.
12. Hagness SCT, Taflove A, Bridges JE. Two-dimensional FDTD analysis of a pulsed microwave confocal system for breast cancer detection: fixed-focus and antenna-array sensors. EEE Trans Biomed Eng. 1998;45:1470–9.
13. Fear ECL, Li X, Hagness SH, Stuchly MA. Confocal microwave imaging for breast cancer detection: localization of tumors in three dimensions. IEEE Trans Biomed Eng. 2002;49(8):812–22.
14. Hand JWH, Hynynen K, Shivastava PN, Saylor TK. Methods of external hyperthermic heating. Berlin: Springer; 1990.
15. Wust PH, Hildebrandt B, Sreenivasa G, Rau B, Gellermann J, Riess H, Felix R, Schlag PM. Hyperthermia in combined treatment of cancer. Lancet Oncol. 2002;3:487–97.
16. Kruger RAK, Kopecky K, Aisen AM, Reinecke DR, Kruger GA, Kiser Jr WL. Thermoacoustic CT with radio-waves: a medical imaging paradigm. Radiology. 1999;211(1):275–8.

Part III

New Therapeutic Options
for Focal Therapy of PCa

Focal or Multifocal Therapy in Prostate Cancer: New Technologies and Strategies

7

Stephanie Guillaumier, Mark Emberton, and Hashim U. Ahmed

Contents

7.1 Introduction

New surgical techniques are continuously being developed in the field of prostate cancer, more so with the ever-increasing interest in minimally invasive techniques to treat solid organ cancers. This has been triggered by the current state of play with treating a disease that has a long natural history in which the benefits and risks of radical therapy are not quite right. In other words, whole-gland radical therapy or radiotherapy can cause significant complications that are a direct result of damage to surrounding structures, including erectile dysfunction (30–70 %), urinary incontinence (5–20 %) and bowel toxicity (5–10 %) [1, 2]. Focal therapy aims to reduce the complication profile by focusing the therapy to the cancer lesion and preserving surrounding tissues, thus improving functional outcome.

S. Guillaumier (✉) • M. Emberton • H.U. Ahmed
Division of Surgery and Interventional Sciences, University College London, London, UK
e-mail: Stephanie.Guillaumier@uclh.nhs.uk;
mark.emberton@uclh.nhs.uk; hashim.ahmed@ucl.ac.uk

© Springer International Publishing Switzerland 2015
S. Thüroff, C.G. Chaussy (eds.), *Focal Therapy of Prostate Cancer:
An Emerging Strategy for Minimally Invasive, Staged Treatment*,
DOI 10.1007/978-3-319-14160-2_7

Improvements in understanding about the biology of prostate cancer as well as huge strides in functional imaging and image-guided biopsy techniques have given rise to more accurate localisation and characterisation of prostate cancer lesions. This has led to a paradigm shift in prostate cancer treatment towards tissue-preserving focal approaches using high-intensity focused ultrasound, electroporation and photodynamic therapy. Focal therapy involves treating just the areas of prostate harbouring cancer and, by doing so, minimising the damage caused to collateral structures such as neurovascular bundles, external urinary sphincter, bladder neck and rectum. In this chapter, we review the rationale for and early results of focal therapy.

7.2   The Index Lesion

Prostate cancer is a multifocal disease. Traditionally, the heterogeneity of the disease has had to be treated with whole-gland therapies, such as radical prostatectomy or radiotherapy, because of the inability to detect and localise individual foci of disease reliably. With the advent of PSA screening, more men are diagnosed with prostate cancer at an earlier stage, when this is still localised. A significant proportion of unifocal or unilateral disease – between 20 and 40 % approximately – has been reported. As a result, focal therapy – with either unifocal ablation or hemiablation strategies – has been suggested as a means to offer men control of their cancer without the genitourinary side effects associated with radical whole-gland therapies (Figs. 7.1 and 7.2).

Recently, the concept of the index lesion has come to the fore. Many physicians now believe that the largest tumour volume usually harbours the highest Gleason

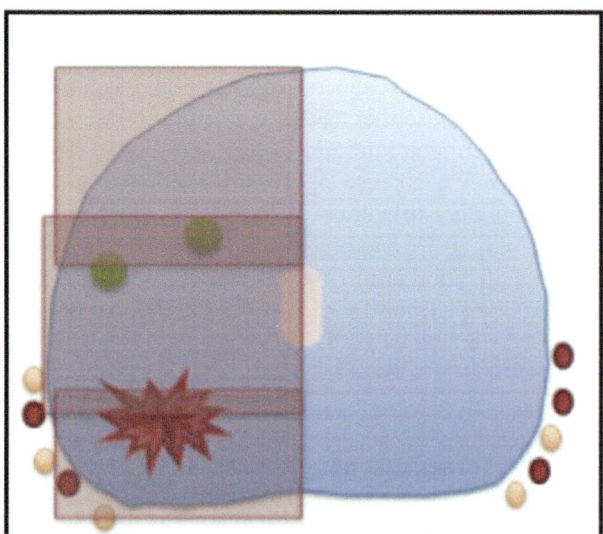

Fig 7.1 Schematic diagram showing hemiablation

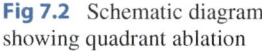
Fig 7.2 Schematic diagram showing quadrant ablation

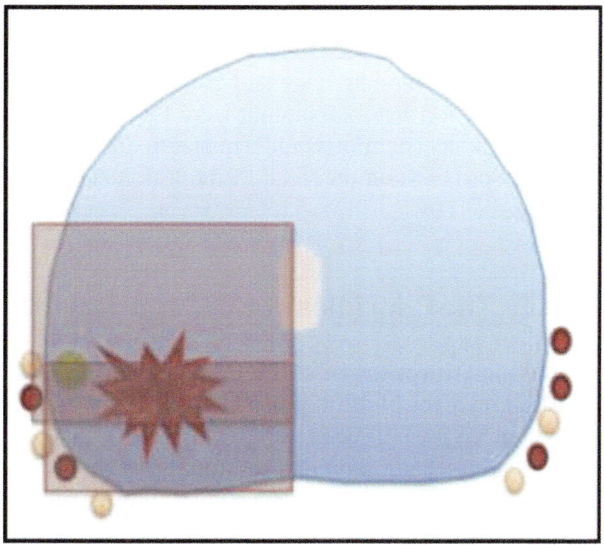

grade – termed the index tumour – and this is the primary determinant of progression of the disease. Although this is often accompanied by secondary tumours, on average 2–3, these on the whole do not progress.

The evidence for this comes from a number of sources. Ohori et al.'s study analysed 1,000 retropubic prostatectomy specimens from men diagnosed with early-stage prostate cancer. Eighteen per cent of lesions were unilateral. Any extracapsular extension that was present was associated with the largest intra-prostatic cancer lesion. This implies that effectively treating the index lesion would destroy the tumour burden that is likely to result in invasive or metastatic disease [3].

This was supported by another study by Karavitakis et al. They showed that although 79 % of cases were multifocal, when pathological features of poor prognosis were present – Gleason $\geq$7, extracapsular invasion and seminal vesicle invasion – they normally resided in the index lesion. Of 170 satellite lesions, 86 % had a total volume of <0.5 ml and 99 % had a Gleason score of <6 [4].

Genomic studies have also supported the index lesion hypothesis. One of the genetic changes present in prostate cancer is the translocation of gene *TMPRSS2-ERG*. This results in overexpression of the ERG transcription factor which promotes proliferation, one of the hallmarks of malignancy. One study carried out by Furusato et al. demonstrated that the RMPRSS-ERG fusions are predominantly found in the index lesion [5].

Men usually present with two or more distinct lesions of cancer within the prostate. Most of the tumour burden is normally contained within one of these foci. Tumour volume is strongly associated with grade, and because of its potential for malignancy, the lesion with the highest tumour volume has been labelled the index lesion, as described by Wise et al. They demonstrated that the volume of the largest tumour, Gleason patterns 4 and 5 as well as lymphovascular invasion predicted progression of prostate cancer [6].

Further evidence on tumour volume being key to progression potential of prostate lesions of emerges from several sources. Investigators have shown that, after accounting for tumour stage and grade, the minimum threshold tumour volume of the index lesion and total tumour were 1.3 and 2.5 cm^3 [7–9]. In unifocal lesions, the mean tumour volume would equate to the total tumour volume and therefore increase progression potential of the lesion. This further supports the index lesion hypothesis [10].

7.3   The Principles of HIFU and Sonablate 500

Ultrasound waves can be of low or high intensity. High-intensity focused ultrasound (HIFU) involves high-intensity ultrasound waves focused on a single point, aimed at a targeted area of the prostate. The temperature at this focal point will rise, causing protein denaturation and destruction of lipid membranes, resulting in coagulative necrosis of the tissue. This allows delivery of treatment to a discrete volume of tissue [11].

The Sonablate®500 (Focus Surgery, Indianapolis, IN, USA) is one of two commercially available transrectal devices that are used to treat prostate cancer. The other is the Ablatherm® Device (Edap-Technomed, Lyon, France).

The Sonablate®500 system has a rectal probe containing a transducer, which has combined imaging and therapeutic roles. It operates with a frequency of 4 MHz. After each pulse of treatment cycle, the transducer takes an imaging shot, allowing visualisation of the treatment effect. Degassed chilled water, at 17–20 °C, is pumped through the whole system to prevent build-up of heat with subsequent rectal wall injury (Sonachill®). The area of treatment can be targeted precisely by adjusting the focal length of the transducer, which is set at 3 or 4 cm focal lengths.

The power intensity delivered at each focal length can be altered according to the greyscale changes seen with each pulse (visually directed HIFU). These greyscale changes, termed 'Uchida' changes, are due to steam build-up in the targeted area (gas microbubbles) causing a cavitation effect and giving an indication as to cell kill. The Sonablate®500 system allows focal, zonal and hemiablation of the prostate gland. The system utilises what is known as Tissue Change Monitoring. This is a quantitative software module designed exclusively for the Sonablate 500 that monitors real-time tissue changes during HIFU therapy. It provides feedback on the status of ablative therapy in real time so the physician knows exactly what is happening to the prostatic tissue. The TCM works by sending a radio-frequency signal to a treatment site prior to delivery of HIFU and then another signal sent after delivery of HIFU in the same treatment site. The software calculates the change that took place, displaying it on screen. It quantifies tissue changes based on comparison of radio-frequency ultrasound pulse-echo signals at each treatment site (Fig. 7.3).

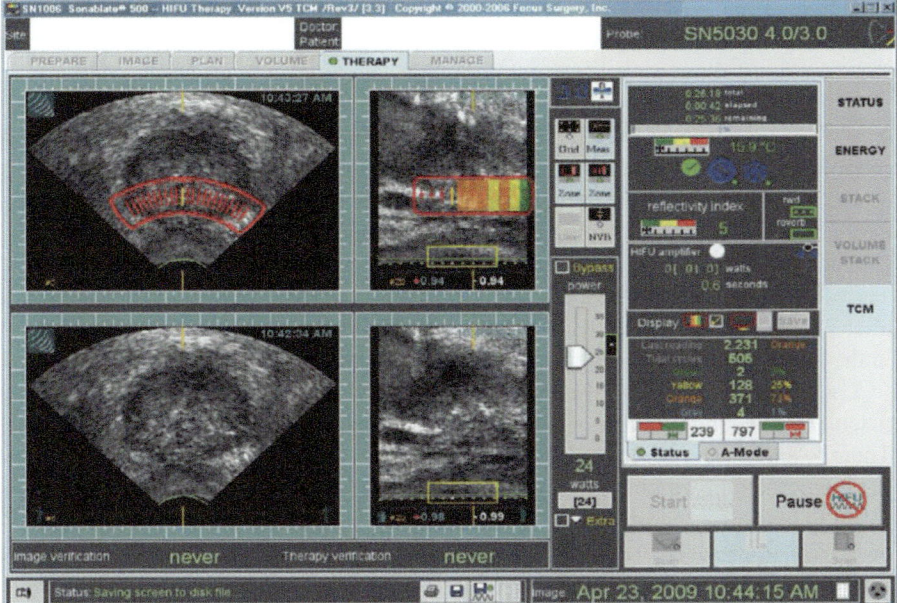

Fig 7.3 Sonablate 500 TCM monitor screen displaying real-time imaging with baseline imaging simultaneously

7.4   Focal Therapy with HIFU

Ahmed et al. published results on their series of high-intensity focused ultrasound hemiablation. From a total of 20 men, 89 % achieved the trifecta status of pad-free, leak-free continence, erections sufficient for intercourse and cancer control at 12 months [12]. A year later, the same group of investigators published their results on another series whereby 42 men received focal high-intensity focused ultrasound delivered to all known cancer lesions with a margin of normal tissue. The results demonstrated that 95 % had no evidence of disease on multiparametric MRI at 12 months. Of 35 men with good baseline erections, 89 % had erections sufficient for penetration 12 months after HIFU therapy. All 38 men with no urinary incontinence at baseline were leak-free and pad-free by 9 months [13]. The same group's prospective academic registry demonstrates that of 509 men undergoing focal HIFU therapy, only 17 % required redo-HIFU, 1 % had salvage radiotherapy and another 1 % went on to be treated with radiotherapy [14].

Another series on focal high-intensity focused ultrasound comes from Muto et al. The results show that 76.6 % of those receiving focal HIFU were biopsy-negative at 12 months and the 2-year biochemical disease-free status rates for the patients at low and intermediate risk 83.3 and 53.6 %, respectively, in patients with focal therapy [15].

Uchida et al. published their long-term results of high-intensity focused ultrasound in localised prostate cancer in 2009. A total of 517 men were included, having a median follow-up period of 24 months. The biochemical disease-free rate in all patients at 5 years was 72 %. In the low-, intermediate- and high-risk group, this was 84, 64 and 53 %, respectively. 28.9 % of patients that had good erectile function preoperatively were reported to have erectile dysfunction post-HIFU treatment [16].

Inoue et al. published their long-term outcomes on 137 patients with T1-2 prostate cancer and a median follow-up of 36 months. They were treated with HIFU (Sonablate®500). They report that no patients proceeded to receiving adjuvant therapy within the follow-up period. The median PSA nadir was 0.07 ng/ml and occurred after 2 months. The 5-year disease-free survival rate was 78 % and 91, 81 and 62 % in the low-, intermediate- and high-risk group, respectively [17].

Encouraging data has also been published by Crouzet et al., with the Edap machine. Their multicentre study included 803 patients from six French centres. Their 5- and 7-year biochemical survival rates for the low-risk group were 83 and 75 %, respectively, and for the intermediate-risk group were 72 and 63 %, respectively. They also reported that at 8 years, the overall survival rate was 89 %, metastasis-free survival was 97 % and cancer-specific survival was 99 % [18]. Similarly, Blana et al. reported on 163 patients with a 4.8 ± 1.2 years of follow-up. The actuarial biochemical survival rate at 5 years was 75 % and disease-free survival rate, also at 5 years, was 66 %. Only 12 % of patients progress to salvage treatment. Of these, 92.7 % had negative biopsy after treatment and 86.4 % achieved a PSA nadir of <1 ng/ml [19].

7.5   Photodynamic Therapy

Photodynamic therapy uses a photosensitising drug that is activated in the presence of oxygen, by light of a specific wavelength, after a period of time (drug-light interval). The drug can be available in topical, oral or intravenous form. The photosensitiser is initially in a stable form, known as ground state. Light of a specific wavelength will transform it to a higher unstable energy state, the singlet state. Being unstable, the photosensitiser can release energy in one of three ways: emission of light, emission of heat or conversion to an intermediate energy state, the triplet state. It can then return to a stable ground state.

The photosensitiser either produces hydroxyl and superoxide radicals (type 1 reaction) or converts to molecular tissue oxygen to form singlet oxygen (type 2 reaction). The singlet oxygen will, in turn, react with lipids, protein and nucleic acids in the cell, leading to both functional and structural damage with subsequent cell death. Hydroxyl and superoxide radicals, in their own right, are also directly responsible for cell death. Drug, light and oxygen must all be present and exceed a specific threshold, for photodynamic therapy to occur.

There are various types of photosensitisers, broadly differentiated into two categories: vascular activated or tissue activated. Those activated within the vasculature do so within a few minutes of intravenous administration and exhibit rapid clearance. This gives them a short drug-light interval. Tissue-activated photosensitisers are activated when sufficient concentration within the tissue target is reached. This may take from several hours to days, hence a delayed drug-light interval. This type of photosensitisers can accumulate in the eyes and skin. Ambient light can activate them and cause a sunburn-like reaction [20].

Types of intravenous photosensitisers include the following:

- Hematoporphyrin derivative (HpD)
- WST-09 (Palladium bacteriopheophorhide, Tookad)
- WST-11 (Palladium bacteriopheophorbide)
- Porfirmer derivative (Photofrin)
- Mesotetrahydroxyphenylchlorin (mTHPF, Foscan)
- Motexafin lutetium

Oral photosensitiser

- ALA (aminolevulinic acid)

Photoradiation was initially used to treat superficial conditions such as lupus vulgaris in the nineteenth century. The first attempt at using phototherapy for human tumours was carried out in 1903 by Tappenier and Jesionek. More recently, in the 1970s, it was used on cutaneous or subcutaneous malignant lesions. In 1978, Dougherty et al. published data on PDT being used on solid tumours, which included prostate and breast. They used haematoporphyrin hydrochloride and red light. One patient with prostate cancer was treated with HPD, with 'complete response', defined as the disappearance of measurable of palpable tumour within a treated field [21].

Photodynamic therapy of the prostate is performed in the lithotomy position under general anaesthesia. Protection to skin and eyes is necessary. This should continue up to a few hours for vascular-activated photosensitisers and up to 6 weeks for tissue-activated ones. A urinary catheter is placed intraoperatively. The photosensitiser is given prior to hospital admission or on the same day as the procedure. Light is produced by laser and delivered by optical fibres. The laser fibres are positioned in the prostate using transrectal ultrasound and a perineal template.

In the prostate, the procedure was first carried out in canines, as this is the closest anatomical model to the human prostate. Huang et al. carried out laparotomies in five dogs. Light at 50–300 J/cm at 150 mW/cm and 763 mm was delivered to the prostate to activate the vascular-activated photosensitiser, padoporfin (Tookad) IV (1 mg.kg b.w.). Varying treatment protocols and light doses on each dog were used to achieve different amounts of necrosis and treatment effect. Contrast-enhanced MRI at 7 days post-PDT showed enhancement corresponding to pathological areas of necrosis. Contrast-enhanced MRI was shown to be superior to diffusion-weighted and T2 images.

The first formal clinical trial was conducted by Nathan et al. This group delivered photodynamic therapy using mesotetrahydroxyphenylchlorin (mTHPC – Foscan) in

14 men, using high light doses in 13 men MRI or contrast-enhanced CT post-procedure showing necrosis in 91 % of the gland. PSA decreased in 9 patients and had no malignancy in post-treatment. Complications included acute urinary retention (3/14), urinary incontinence (2/14) and recto-urethral fistula (1/14). The fistula occurred after a rectal biopsy following the treatment. A further pilot study was conducted by this group, again using mTHPC. Six patients were treated, all of which were found to have residual tumour on biopsy. Four received a second treatment with PDT; one opted for active surveillance and the other, radiotherapy [22].

The palladium pheophorbide photosensitisers padoporfin (WST-09 Tookad®) and padeliporfin (WST-11 Tookad® Soluble) are vascular-acting PDT agents. Trachtenberg et al. used WST-09 (Tookad®) as vascular-targeted photodynamic therapy (VTP) for whole-gland prostate ablation to treat men with radio-recurrent localised prostate cancer. Twenty-eight patients received varying light doses. A complete response was seen in 8 out of 13 patients. This was determined by performing prostate biopsies at 6 months. The minimum light dose required to cause necrosis was 23 J/cm^3 in 90 % of the prostate. Treatment response was assessed by gadolinium-enhanced MRI after 1 week. Avascular lesions on MRI correlated with histopathological fibrosis. Sixty per cent of those who received the minimum light dose at 2 mg/kg drug dose had no residual disease on biopsy [23]. Systemic toxicity was observed with padoporfin (WST-09): cardiovascular events and subclinical hepatotoxicity secondary to intraoperative hypotension. For this reason, WST-11 Tookad® Soluble was developed. This is a water-soluble version of the drug, known as padeliporfin.

More recently, Moore et al. published their data on 85 patients treated with Tookad® Soluble. Overall, 74 % had negative biopsies at 6 months and the mean percentage of gland necrosis was 78 %. Of the group that received 4 mg/kg of Tookad® Soluble at 200 J/cm, 83 % were found to have negative biopsies at 6 months with the mean percentage of necrosis of targeted prostate tissue being 88 %. They found that 4 mg/kg at 200 J/cm gave the optimal treatment conditions for good short-term efficacy [24].

These studies demonstrate that photodynamic therapy with Tookad® Soluble is well tolerated and shows good short-term efficacy. It can be carried out in a single clinical session as a minimally invasive procedure. PDT is a repeatable procedure and does not exclude patients from further treatments. Positioning of the needles is relatively straightforward. As this is done transperineally, it allows access to the anterior of the prostate gland, inaccessible to certain treatment modalities such as high-intensity focused ultrasound. It is one of the focal treatment options for both primary and salvage localised prostate cancer. Lesion formation is highly dependent on drug and light dose.

There are, however, various limitations to photodynamic ablation as focal therapy for prostate cancer. Treatment planning is based on histopathology and MRI preoperatively, whereas the real-time feedback intraoperatively is ultrasound. Gland deformation during the procedure occurs in part due to the presence of the rectal probe and in part due to the swelling subsequent to transperineal needle insertion. Currently there is no real-time feedback of treatment effect during the delivery of

PDT. A randomised controlled trial of VTP focal therapy versus active surveillance is currently ongoing recruiting very low-risk patients (NCT01726894).

7.6   Irreversible Electroporation

Irreversible electroporation (IRE) is a novel technique, where tissue is ablated through its nonthermal effects. Electroporation involves a significant increase in the electrical conductivity across a cell membrane, by an externally applied electric field. The high-energy direct current causes the lipid bilayer in the cell membrane to lose its integrity, creating nanopores. These nanopores increase the permeability of the cell membrane, losing cellular homeostasis, resulting in subsequent cell death. This phenomenon is dynamic and depends on the electric field strength and tissue properties [25].

A preliminary experimental IRE trial was carried out in a healthy canine and two human cancerous prostates by Neal et al. The electrical parameters to predict treatment stimulations were measured. The prostates were then resected 5 h, 3 weeks and 4 weeks post-IRE. The lesions were correlated with the numerical simulations to determine the effective threshold of the IRE electric field. The results showed that lesions were produced in all subjects. IRE pulses cause an increase in tissue conductivity from 0.285 to 0.927 S/m. The effective average prostate electric field threshold was found to be $1,072 \pm 119$ V/cm. Histological analysis of the human prostates showed complete central necrosis with variable tissue effects beyond the margin of treatment area [26].

Tsivian et al. have published their data on a study carried out on 12 male Beagle dogs using low-energy direct current (NanoKnife™ LEDC). Three 19G monopolar electrodes were placed on each side of the prostate via the transperineal approach under transrectal ultrasound guidance using a triangular probe array. The electrodes were placed at a median distance of 0.55–0.66 cm from the capsule, urethra and rectum. All the dogs were potent postoperatively. Pathological analysis revealed inflammatory changes in the ablation zone at 7 days, which was replaced by fibrosis at 30 days. Microscopic examination showed no histological injury to the capsule, urethra, rectal wall or nerve structures [27].

A pilot study was carried out by Valerio et al. on 45 patients who received IRE, 34 as primary therapy and 11 as salvage treatment. Three men had high-risk disease whilst 31 and 11 men had intermediate- and low-risk disease, respectively. Twenty-eight patients had available follow-up and all achieved urinary continence whilst of the 25 men that were potent preoperatively, 96 % maintained their potency [28]. Ongoing studies will further evaluate the clinical utility of focal IRE (NCT01726894).

Conclusion

Patients diagnosed with prostate cancer are faced with an overwhelming array of possible treatments depending on their disease. Although radical whole-gland therapies such as radical prostatectomy and radiotherapies are still the mainstay of treatment, new surgical innovations have emerged and been revisited over the last couple of decades. Being minimally invasive, they may be viewed in more acceptable light to both patients and surgeon than radical treatments. Focus on the quality of life of patients in the postoperative period has instigated a surge of interest in both minimally invasive operative techniques as well as focal therapy. Certainly, studies on HIFU, cryotherapy and PDT, although in their infancy, seem to demonstrate that the short-term cancer control is comparable to other therapies and their profile of genitourinary complications is less. More long-term data is necessary to further increase our knowledge on the application of these novel surgical techniques.

References

1. Sanda MG, Dunn RL, Beyth RJ, Neuberger MM, et al. Screening for prostate cancer: a systematic review and meta-analysis of randomised controlled trials. BMJ. 2010;341:c4543.
2. Wilt TJ, MacDonald R, Rutks I, et al. Systematic review: comparative effectiveness and harms of treatments for clinically localized prostate cancer. Ann Intern Med. 2008;148:435–48.
3. Ohori M. Multiple cancers in the prostate. Morphologic features of clinically recognized vs incidental tumours. Cancer. 1992;70:2312–8.
4. Karavitakis M. Tumour focality in prostate cancer: implications for focal therapy. Nat Rec Clin Oncol. 2011;8(1):223–7.
5. Furusato B, Gao CL, Ravindranath L, et al. Mapping of TMPRSS2-ERG fusions in the context of multi-focal prostate cancer. Mod Pathol. 2008;21:67–75.
6. Wise AM, Stamey TA, McNeal JE, Clayton JL. Morphologic and clinical significance of mul-tifocal prostate cancers in radical prostatectomy specimens. Urology. 2002;60:264–9.
7. Wolters T, Roobol MJ, van Leeuwen PJ, et al. A critical analysis of the tumor volume threshold for clinically insignificant prostate cancer using a data set of a randomized screening trial. J Urol. 2011;185:121–5.
8. Van der Kwast TH. The trade-off between sensitivity and specificity of clinical protocols for identification of insignificant prostate cancer. Eur Urol. 2012;62:469–71.
9. Fuchsjager MH, Pucar D, Zelefsky MJ, et al. Predicting post-external beam radiation therapy PSA relapse of prostate cancer using pretreatment MRI. Int J Radiat Oncol Biol Phys. 2010;78:743–50.
10. Ahmed HU, Arya M, Freeman A, Emberton M. Do low-grade and low-volume prostate can-cers bear the hallmarks of malignancy? Lancet Oncol. 2012;13(11):e509–17. doi:10.1016/S1470-2045(12)70388-1.
11. Tsakiris P, Thüroff S, de la Rosette J, Chaussy C. Transrectal high-intensity focused ultrasound devices: a critical appraisal of the available evidence. J Endourol. 2008;22(2):221–9.
12. Ahmed HU, Freeman A, Kirkham A, Sahu M, Scott R, Allen C, Can der Meulen J, Emberton M. Focal therapy for localised prostate cancer: a phase I/II trial. J Urol. 2011;185:1246–55.
13. Ahmed HU, Hindley RG, Dickinson L, Freeman A, Sahu M, Scott R, Allen C, Van der Meulen J, Emberton M. Focal therapy for localised unifocal and multifocal prostate cancer: a prospec-tive development study. Lancet Oncol. 2012. doi:10.1016/S1470-2045(12)0121-3.
14. Guillaumier S, Dickinson L, Stone H, McCartan N, Thiruvel M, Hindley RG, Emberton M, Ahmed HU. High-intensity focussed ultrasound in the treatment of localised prostate cancer: focal salvage transition rates. J Urol. 2014;191(4):e714. doi: 10.1016/j.juro.2014.02.1960.
15. Muto S, Yoshii T, Saito K, Kamiyama Y, Ide H, Horie S. Focal therapy with high-intensity-focused ultrasound in the treatment of localized prostate cancer. Jpn J Clin Oncol. 2008;38(3):192–9. doi:10.1093/jjco/hym173. Epub 2008 Feb 15.

16. Uchida T, Shoji S, Nakano M, Hongo S, Nitta M, Murota A, et al. Transrectal high-intensity focused ultrasound for the treatment of localized prostate cancer: eight-year experience. Int J Urol. 2009;16:881–6.
17. Inoue YGK, Goto K, Hayashi T, Hayashi M. Transrectal high-intensity focused ultrasound for treatment of localized prostate cancer. Int J Urol. 2011. doi:10.1111/j.1442-2042.2011.02739.x.
18. Crouzet S, Rebillard X, Chevallier D, Rischmann P, Pasticier G, Garcia G, et al. Multicentric oncologic outcomes of high-intensity focused ultrasound for localized prostate cancer in 803 patients. Eur Urol. 2010;58:559–66.
19. Blana A, Rogenhofer S, Ganzer R, Lunz JC, Schostak M, Wieland WF, et al. Eight years' experience with high-intensity focused ultrasonography for treatment of localized prostate cancer. Urology. 2008;72:1329–33.
20. Moore CM, Hoh I, Bown S, Emberton M. Does photodynamic therapy have the necessary attributes to become a future treatment for organ-confined prostate cancer? BJU Int. 2005;96:754–8.
21. Dougherty T, Kaufman J, Goldfarb A, Weishaupt K, Boyle D, Mittleman A. Photoradiation therapy for the treatment of malignant tumors. Cancer Res. 1978;38:2628–35.
22. Nathan T, Whitelaw D, Chang S, Lees W, Ripley P, Payne H, et al. Photodynamic therapy for prostate cancer recurrence after radiotherapy: a phase I study. J Urol. 2002;168:1427–32.
23. Trachtenburg J, Weersink R, Davidson S, Haider M, Bogaards A, Gertner M, et al. Vascular-targeted photodynamic therapy (padoporfin, WST09) for recurrent prostate cancer after failure of external beam radiotherapy: a study of escalating light doses. BJU Int. 2008;102:556–62.
24. Moore C, Nathan T, Lees W, Freeman A, Emberton M, Bown S. Photodynamic therapy using meso tetra hydroxyl phenyl chlorin (mTHPC) in early prostate cancer. Lasers Surg Med. 2006;385:356–63.
25. Leveille R, Pease K, Salas N. Emerging needle ablation technology in urology. Curr Opin Urol. 2014;24(1):98–103.
26. Neal R, Millar J, Kavnoudias H, Boyce P, Rosenfeldt F, Pham A, et al. In vivo characterization and numerical simulation of prostate properties for non-thermal irreversible electroporation ablation. Prostate. 2014;74(5):458–68.
27. Tsivian M, Polascik T. Bilateral focal ablation of prostate tissue using low-energy direct current (LEDC): a preclinical canine study. BJU Int. 2013;112(4):526–30.
28. Valerio M, Stricker PD, Ahmed HU, Dickinson L, Ponsky L, Shnier R, et al. Initial assessment of safety and clinical feasibility of irreversible electroporation in the focal treatment of prostate cancer. Prostate Cancer Prostatic Dis. 2014;17(4):343–7. doi: 10.1038/pcan.2014.33.

How to Create Evidence for Focal PCa Therapy Research? HIFU Focal Hemiablation as Non-invasive Therapeutic Option

8

Roman Ganzer

Contents

8.1   Introduction

The intention of focal therapy of prostate cancer is to offer the patient a partial treatment of prostate containing only the areas of significant cancer. The goal is a reduction of potential side effects of radical treatment. These side effects are typically caused by collateral damage of anatomical structures adjacent to the prostate, such as the urethral sphincter, the erectile nerves, the bladder neck and the rectum. The need to create more evidence of focal therapy strategies is illustrated against the background of the growing evidence of prostate cancer overtreatment and the related side effects. According to a recent review summarising the situation of overdiagnosis and overtreatment, Loeb et al. showed that overtreatment is estimated to be present in a range of 5–46.8 % in published radical prostatectomy series [1].

R. Ganzer
Department of Urology, University of Leipzig, Leipzig, Germany
e-mail: roman.ganzer@me.com

© Springer International Publishing Switzerland 2015
S. Thüroff, C.G. Chaussy (eds.), *Focal Therapy of Prostate Cancer:
An Emerging Strategy for Minimally Invasive, Staged Treatment*,
DOI 10.1007/978-3-319-14160-2_8

87

Although outcome of radical prostatectomy has improved over the last years, it may still be associated with significant morbidity even in the hands of high-volume surgeons. In a series of 380 preoperatively potent patients, Shikanov et al. showed that the trifecta (continence, potency and undetectable PSA) was achieved in only 44 % of patients 24 months following nerve-sparing robotic-assisted radical prostatectomy (RALP) [2].

8.2   Strategies and Technologies for Focal Prostate Treatment

Despite a growing number of studies and case series in the literature, there is no clear definition of the ideal way how to perform focal prostate cancer treatment. Different treatment regimens have been described. They include targeting of a radiographic and biopsy-proven index lesion, but also a sextant, a three-quarter, a hockey-stick and a hemiablation approach. The future goal will be to eradicate only significant cancer foci, which might be feasible once the ideal imaging or cancer detection modality has been found. To our knowledge, there has been no successful attempt of a partial radical prostatectomy. Partial ablation of the prostate however has been described with different technologies. These include cryotherapy, high-intensity focussed ultrasound (HIFU), laserablation, photodynamic therapy (PDT) and irreversible electroporation (IRE). Today most evidence is available for cryotherapy and HIFU. Therefore, the European Association of Urology (EAU) guidelines mention both these technologies as experimental options for focal therapy. As we have gained experience with HIFU for many years, we will focus on that modality in this chapter.

HIFU works by ultrasound that is administered by a rectal probe and focussed on a target point. This results in a combined thermal and mechanical effect (cavitation) leading to the immediate formation of a sharply confined coagulation necrosis in the shape of a cigar. Currently there are two HIFU devices commercially available on the market: the Ablatherm (EDAP-TMS, Vaulx-en-Velin, France) and the Sonablate (Focus Surgery Inc., Indianapolis, IN, USA). We recently published the outcome of a consecutive patient series of 538 patients following full-gland HIFU. The median follow-up of 8.1 years (range 2.1–14 years) was the longest follow-up in current literature [3]. The biochemical-free survival rates, as defined according to the Phoenix criteria, were 81 and 61 % at 5 and 10 years, respectively. Typical side effects of HIFU are the formation of secondary bladder neck obstruction, with a rate of 28.3 % in our series. Continence outcome is favourable, but due to the heterogeneity of treated patients and different outcome criteria in published studies, there cannot be drawn any conclusion from the literature if full-gland HIFU offers any advantage for potency preservation compared to standard treatment options. The recommendations for full-gland HIFU are conflicting within European urologic associations. It is recommended for selected patients by the French and Italian guidelines but is still considered experimental by the European and German guidelines.

8.3   The Role of HIFU in Focal Therapy

HIFU is a promising tool for focal prostate treatment for different reasons. It allows for precise treatment of a targeted volume, and it is relatively minimally invasive and can be offered as an outpatient procedure under spinal anaesthesia.

The idea behind treating only one lobe of the prostate is to leave the neurovascular bundle on the contralateral side of the prostate completely untouched. Furthermore, it is assumed that the rate of secondary bladder neck obstruction will be significantly lower compared to full-gland ablation. The first publication of HIFU hemiablation came from [4]. In their series of 70 patients, they classified 29 patients as having unilateral disease as determined by multiregional biopsies. In these patients, only the peripheral zone of one lobe and half of the ipsilateral transitional zone were treated. The remaining patients underwent whole-gland ablation. Twelve months following treatment, 77 % of patients had a negative biopsy. According to the ASTRO criteria, biochemical-free survival rates were 83 and 54 % of patients in the low- and intermediate-risk group, respectively. Of 52 patients that were continent before HIFU, 49 remained continent after treatment. However, the authors did not differentiate between the whole-gland group and the focal group. Also, they did not present outcome data on potency [4].

In 2011, more detailed outcome data from a prospective phase I/II approval trial were published by Ahmed et al. Unilateral prostate carcinoma was identified in 20 patients by means of multiparametric MRI in combination with transperineal mapping biopsy. Patients underwent HIFU hemiablation and were followed up for 12 months; 19/20 patients had erections sufficient for intercourse, 90 % were pad-free and 17/19 patients had no evidence of cancer on control biopsy. Eighty-nine per cent of all patients achieved the trifecta of continence, potency and cancer control at 12 months [5]. Later, the same group developed more advanced treatment strategies including multifocal targeting of prostate cancer foci as will be illustrated in a different chapter in this book.

8.4   Study Endpoints of Focal Therapy Studies

The definition of study endpoints and outcome criteria for focal therapy studies is a challenge. There have been numerous recommendations by panels and expert groups. However, they are in many aspects conflicting. The biggest difficulty is the definition of an oncologic endpoint. Due to the natural history of slowly growing prostate cancer in low- and intermediate-risk patients, cancer-specific survival cannot be used as an endpoint as follow-up periods of far more than 10 years would be required to obtain evidence. Furthermore, prostate-specific antigen (PSA) kinetics following focal therapy have not yet been thoroughly studied and understood. The interpretation of PSA in patients with a partially ablated prostate is difficult, as there will be ablated cancer tissue next to untreated benign prostate hyperplasia and potentially untreated insignificant cancer. It is also unknown, if PSA kinetics are specifically characteristic for different focal therapy technologies. Therefore a biochemical failure definition for patients following focal prostate cancer treatment has yet to be defined. In summary, an early indicator for oncologic efficacy of focal therapy should be based on the result of a control biopsy at 12 months after treatment. In addition to early oncologic outcome, functional results, quality of life and safety should be assessed by means of validated questionnaires.

In an attempt to obtain consensus on design of focal therapy trials, an expert panel summarised options of 48 focal therapy experts in 2014 and defined strict criteria [6]. They defined the first oncologic endpoint as focal ablation of clinically significant disease (tumour >0.5 cc with negative biopsy at 12 months). PSA should not be included as an endpoint. There was an agreement that multiparametric magnetic resonance imaging (mpMRI) is an accurate tool to identify intraprostatic significant disease as the ultimate tool for non-invasive cancer detection is still missing. It was considered that its potential is in excluding patients with aggressive cancers (Gleason score $4+3=7$ and higher) from focal treatment but that a biopsy-proven lesion does not necessarily have to be visible of mpMRI. A systematic and targeted follow-up biopsy was recommended at 6–12 months following treatment. There was no agreement on a biochemical failure definition. Recommendations for future study duration were 18–36 months for phase 2 single arm studies and 3–5 years for phase 3 prospective comparative trials.

8.5   Practical Aspects for Focal Therapy Trials

When designing a focal therapy trial, it should be considered that it is not too much in conflict with daily clinical practice and the expectations of patients and their referring physicians. The ideal trial design would be a prospective randomised controlled trial of a large patient number and a long follow-up period comparing focal therapy with either active surveillance or radical treatment. Such a trial is difficult to generate due to many reasons. Most important, a statistically significant oncologic endpoint between both groups would only be expected after a follow-up period of many years and a large number of patients. In addition, it is questionable whether the majority of eligible patients would be willing to accept randomisation between two options. This concern might be illustrated by the fact that radical prostatectomy is the only treatment option that has been randomised against another approach (watchful waiting) [7]. There are no other publications of successful randomisations between radical prostatectomy and radiotherapy or other treatment options.

For these reasons we designed a phase II study of HIFU hemiablation for patients with unilateral prostate cancer that refuse to undergo active surveillance (HEMI study). The inclusion criteria are shown in Table 8.1. Our intention was a trial design that includes diagnostic procedures that are compatible with the routine of German university hospitals and referring urologists. We therefore decided not to use perineal mapping biopsy of the prostate. Our approach to rule out unilateral disease is by a 12-fold randomised biopsy that is combined with an mpMRI performed at least 4 weeks after biopsy. Patients will be followed up every 3 months for 1 year. Table 8.2 gives an example of a follow-up plan that considers oncologic aspects as

Table 8.1 HEMI study – Eligibility criteria

Eligibility criteria	Age >18 years
	Biopsy-proven prostate cancer
	Clinical stages T1c–T2a
	PSA ≤10 ng/ml
	Gleason score ≤7a (3 + 4)
	Unilateral prostate cancer
	Number of positive biopsies <30 % of the total number of biopsies with the largest continuous tumour area <5 mm
	Height of peripheral zone on treatment side on TRUS
	≤30 mm (in treatments with Ablatherm Integrated Imaging)
	≤40 mm (in treatments with Focal One)
	No evidence of significant prostate cancer on contralateral prostate lobe on multiparametric MRI (defined as PI-RADS Scores 4 and 5)
	Thickness of the rectal wall <6 mm on TRUS
	Acceptance of participation in all follow-up visits (during 12 months)

well as safety and quality of life. We defined our primary endpoint as "no initiation of any definitive prostate cancer treatment (radical prostatectomy, radiation, full-gland HIFU, cryotherapy, hormone therapy) within the study period." Besides several secondary endpoints, validated questionnaires are used to assess safety and morbidity: urinary function is assessed by the International Prostate Symptom Score (IPSS) and the short form of the International Consultation on Incontinence Modular Questionnaire (ICIQ-SF). Quality of life is measured with the European Organisation for Research and Treatment of Cancer Quality of Life Questionnaire (EORTC QLQ-30) and erectile function with the short form of the International Index of Erectile Function (IIEF-5) questionnaire. We hypothesise that patients that undergo focal treatment might feel less bothered by anxiety than many patients with untreated cancer. To measure this we included the Hospital Anxiety and Depression Scale (HADS) questionnaire to rule out if there is a decrease in anxiety and psychological burden compared to the situation before treatment. In addition, all treatment-related side effects are measured. As the trial is still enrolling, we cannot present results at this point.

8.6 Future Technical Aspects

In 2013, a new generation of HIFU device (Focal One) was released by EDAP-TMS. Besides some technical refinements, the most important feature is the option to fuse prostate MRI images with the transrectal ultrasound image in real time. The height of the lesions is reduced from a minimum of 19 mm with the Ablatherm Integrated Imaging to 5 mm. These features promise new options of focal prostate cancer treatment and will improve targeting of prostate zones with low anterior-posterior diameter (such as the peripheral zone at the apex). However, data are currently lacking and will have to be generated in order to prove the expected advantages of this device in comparison to previous generations.

Table 8.2 Study plan on "prospective phase II study on focal therapy (hemiablation) of the prostate with high-intensity focussed ultrasound (HIFU)) in patients suitable for active surveillance"

	V1	V2	V3	V4	V5	V6	V7	V8	V9	V10
	Screening		Inclusion	Pretreatment	Treatment	Follow-up	Follow-up	Follow-up	Follow-up	Follow-up
				Day 1	Day 0	Month 1	Month 3	Month 6	Month 9	Month 12
Screening for inclusion/exclusion criteria	✓			✓						
Informed consent	✓		✓	✓						
History	✓					✓	✓	✓	✓	✓
Clinical investigation	✓						✓	✓	✓	✓
Transrectal ultrasound (TRUS)	✓						✓	✓	✓	✓
Multiparametric MRI		✓								
Prostate-specific antigen (PSA)	✓					✓	✓	✓	✓	✓
Urinalysis and urine culture	✓									
Uroflow	✓						✓	✓	✓	✓
12-fold biopsy of the prostate			✓							
Assessment of additional treatment						✓	✓	✓	✓	✓
Charlson comorbidity score	✓									
IPSS			✓			✓	✓	✓	✓	✓
ICIQ-SF			✓				✓	✓	✓	✓
EORTC QLQ 30			✓				✓	✓	✓	✓
IIEF 5			✓				✓	✓	✓	
HADS-D			✓				✓	✓	✓	
HIFU treatment (hemiablation)					✓					
Adverse events (AE)					✓	✓	✓	✓	✓	✓

8.7   Limitations of Focal HIFU

The concept of focal HIFU treatment still has limitations to be mentioned. In a recent study, Shoji et al. could show that there is significant swelling and shift of the prostate during HIFU treatment. This will make real-time intraoperative adjustment of the treatment plan mandatory, once smaller prostate cancer foci will be targeted [8]. A second limitation for all focal treatment approaches in prostate cancer is the difficulty to identify unilateral disease by means of random biopsy only. Isbarn et al. performed a retrospective study in 243 men with only 2/10 positive biopsies on one side, a Gleason score ≤6 and a PSA value of ≤10 ng/ml. Interestingly, two-thirds of these patients had either bilateral or even non-organ-confined disease following radical prostatectomy. This underlines that a random biopsy alone is insufficient to identify patients suitable for hemiablation. Therefore, mpMRI should be combined with random biopsy instead of mapping biopsies in order to rule out significant contralateral disease.

Conclusions

In conclusion, first reports on patient series of HIFU hemiablation demonstrate the feasibility of this concept. Early oncologic results as assessed by control biopsy are promising, but follow-up is still much too short to prove long-term oncologic efficacy. Much of progress in focal therapy may be expected in the next years. This evolution is necessary in order to identify the ideal patient subgroup that benefits from focal therapy. It is important to clarify the subgroup of patients, which might be overtreated and the one which is undertreated and put at risk with focal therapy. In the future, new innovative imaging modalities and methods to assess tumour aggressiveness will be the basis for more refined approaches in focal therapy of prostate cancer. The results of future studies will then be indirectly comparable to those of "historic" studies of patients treated with hemiablation.

References

1. Loeb S, Bjurlin MA, Nicholson J, Tammela TL, Penson DF, Carter HB, Carroll P, Etzioni R. Overdiagnosis and overtreatment of prostate cancer. Eur Urol. 2014;65(6):1046–55. doi:10.1016/j.eururo.2013.12.062. pii: S0302-2838(13)01490-5.
2. Shikanov SA, Zorn KC, Zagaja GP, Shalhav AL. Trifecta outcomes after robotic-assisted laparoscopic prostatectomy. Urology. 2009;74(3):619–23. doi:10.1016/j.urology.2009.02.082. Epub 2009 Jul 9.
3. Ganzer R, Fritsche HM, Brandtner A, Bründl J, Koch D, Wieland WF, Blana A. Fourteen-year oncological and functional outcomes of high-intensity focused ultrasound in localized prostate cancer. BJU Int. 2013;112(3):322–9.
4. Muto S, Yoshii T, Saito K, Kamiyama Y, Ide H, Horie S. Focal therapy with high-intensity-focused ultrasound in the treatment of localized prostate cancer. Jpn J Clin Oncol. 2008;38(3):192–9.
5. Ahmed HU, Freeman A, Kirkham A, Sahu M, Scott R, Allen C, Van der Meulen J, Emberton M. Focal therapy for localized prostate cancer: a phase I/II trial. J Urol. 2011;185(4):1246–54.

6. van den Bos W, Muller BG, Ahmed H, Bangma CH, Barret E, Crouzet S, Eggener SE, Gill IS, Joniau S, Kovacs G, Pahernik S, de la Rosette JJ, Rouvière O, Salomon G, Ward JF, Scardino PT. Focal therapy in prostate cancer: international multidisciplinary consensus on trial design. Eur Urol. 2014;65(6):1078–83. doi:10.1016/j.eururo.2014.01.001. pii: S0302-2838(14)00002-5.
7. Bill-Axelson A, Garmo H, Holmberg L, Johansson JE, Adami HO, Steineck G, Johansson E, Rider JR. Long-term distress after radical prostatectomy versus watchful waiting in prostate cancer: a longitudinal study from the Scandinavian Prostate Cancer Group-4 randomized clinical trial. Eur Urol. 2013;64(6):920–8.
8. Shoji S, Uchida T, Nakamoto M, Kim H, de Castro Abreu AL, Leslie S, Sato Y, Gill IS, Ukimura O. Prostate swelling and shift during high intensity focused ultrasound: implication for targeted focal therapy. J Urol. 2013;190(4):1224–32.

Salvage Focal HIFU

9

Sébastien Crouzet

Contents

9.1 Salvage Focal HIFU After Radiation Therapy

Prostate cancer recurrence after radiation therapy might be cured with different treatment modalities (radical prostatectomy, HIFU, cryotherapy). All whole-gland salvage therapy approaches carry the potential of serious morbidity from the development of urethro-rectal fistula, severe urinary incontinence, and urethral stenosis [1–5].

Focal salvage HIFU (FSH) represents a new therapeutic option with the aim to destroy the recurrent tumor with minimal risk of severe side effects. The initial results of this new treatment approach were recently published [6]. In this trial, 39 patients received focal salvage HIFU therapy for localized recurrence after EBRT (hemiablation, $n = 16$; quadrant ablation, $n = 23$). Patients with multifocal tumor foci underwent index lesion ablation if the untreated areas had ≤1 core with ≤3 mm 3 + 3 Gleason score. A PSA response was observed in 87 % of patients; 44 % of treated patients achieved a PSA nadir <0.5 ng/ml. Of those who achieved a nadir <0.5, the 3-year biochemical-free survival sate (BFSR) (Phoenix criteria) was 63 %. Of those who achieved a nadir >0.5, the 3-year BFSR was 0 %. Two patients developed

S. Crouzet
Urology Department, Edouard Herriot Hospital, Lyon, France
e-mail: Sebastien.crouzet@chu-lyon.fr

© Springer International Publishing Switzerland 2015
S. Thüroff, C.G. Chaussy (eds.), *Focal Therapy of Prostate Cancer:
An Emerging Strategy for Minimally Invasive, Staged Treatment*,
DOI 10.1007/978-3-319-14160-2_9

metastasis and 40 % required salvage androgen deprivation therapy. Twenty-five patients (64 %) were continent (pad-free, leak-free) at the last follow-up. The mean pre-salvage IIEF-15 score decreased from 18 ± 16 to 13 ± 21 after FSH.

More recently, Baco et al. reported the short-term results of hemi-salvage HIFU ablation (HSH) for unilateral recurrent PCa following radiation therapy [7]. Between 2009 and 2012, 48 patients were prospectively enrolled from two European centers. Inclusion criteria were positive MRI and at least one positive biopsy in one lobe after primary radiation therapy without detectable metastases, as determined by bone scan, pelvic CT scan or pelvic MRI.

The mean age was 68.8 ± 6 years and the mean pre-HIFU PSA was 5.2 ± 5.2 ng/ml.

The treatment phase, controlled by the device software, was processed by successive slices (1.7 mm thick) from apex to base. Treatment parameters for HIFU therapy involved a 3-MHZ nominal frequency, a 5-s treatment pulse, and a 4-s shot interval. The necrotic coagulation zone induced by one treatment pulse, termed the elementary lesion, was 1.7 mm in diameter and 19–27 mm in height, depending on prostate AP diameter. A 4-mm security distance was observed at the apex in cases with negative apical biopsy, but some HIFU shots were performed closer to the sphincter in cases with apical invasion. Similarly, treatment included the proximal region of the seminal vesicle in patients with basal tumor invasion of the prostate.

With a median follow-up of 16.3 months, the mean PSA nadir after HSH was 0.69 ± 0.83 ng/ml. Disease progression occurred in 16 patients (35.5 %). Local recurrence was found in the untreated lobe in 4 patients and bilaterally in 4 patients. Six patients developed metastases and 2 had rising PSA without local recurrence or radiologically proven metastasis. Progression-free survival (Phoenix criteria) rates at 12, 18, and 24 months were 83, 64, and 52 %, respectively. No rectal fistula was observed. There were no significant changes in EORTC-QLQ C30 and IPSS scores. A pad-free, leak-free urinary continence status after HSH was attained in 36 of 48 patients (75 %). Four patients (8.3 %) experienced severe post-HSH incontinence. All 4 had a post-EBRT local recurrence involving the apex, and HSH was voluntarily performed without a sphincter safety margin. Three of the 4 did not show disease progression; their PSA values at the last follow-up were 0.12, 0.05, and 0.07 ng/ml. No urethro-rectal fistula were observed. Two patients (4 %) experienced a delayed pubic osteitis that was conservatively managed. There were no statistical significant differences in IPSS and QoL (EORTC-QLQ C30) scores before between baseline and follow-up. A significant decrease in erectile function score was observed (IIEF-5 score), with a median of 7.5–5 at 24-month follow-up. One urethro-rectal fistula occurred and was resolved with urinary and bowel diversion. Sloughing occurred in 18 % of patients and urinary tract infection or epididymitis in 8 %. No osteitis was observed.

The rate of complication reported after focal salvage HIFU for radio-recurrent prostate cancer was substantially lower than those found in published reports of standard salvage treatments. Nguyen et al. evaluated the outcome of salvage radical prostatectomy in 531 patients and found a 4.7 % rate of urethro-rectal fistula, an incontinence rate of 41 %, and an anastomotic stenosis rate of 24 % [8]. In a more recent series of salvage radical prostatectomy, Heidenreich et al. reported a 1 % rate of urethro-rectal fistula and a severe incontinence rate of 20 % [9]. Salvage cryo-therapy was evaluated in 510 patients by Nguyen et al., who found a urethro-rectal fistula rate of 2.6 %, a 36 % rate of severe incontinence, and a 17 % rate of bladder neck strictures [8].

Accurate patient selection is an essential precondition for achieving optimal can-cer control with a focal salvage therapy approach. In theory, the selection process should first exclude patients with infraclinical metastases and then further evaluate only those with small unilateral local recurrences. Detection of occult lymph node and bone metastases is hampered by limitations in current imaging technology and by characteristics of the malignancy that make visualization difficult. Metastases were detected during follow-up in 5 % (2/39) of patients in the Ahmed et al. study [6] and in 12.5 % (6/48) of patients in the Baco et al. study [7].

9.2   Salvage Focal HIFU After Radical Prostatectomy

Therapeutic options for local recurrence following radical prostatectomy are lim-ited. HIFU offers a treatment option when local recurrence can be identified through transrectal ultrasound or MRI and verified by biopsies. After treatment with HIFU, the treated areas showed negative biopsies in 77 %. The PSA nadir averaged 0.2 ng/ml and 66 % of the patients achieved PSA nadir values <0.5 ng/ml. During follow-up of 5 years, 91 % of the patients showed no biochemical progress [10–12].

Conclusion

Focal salvage HIFU is feasible in different clinical situations with less severe morbidity than whole-gland salvage therapies and may preserve pretreatment QoL. Patient selection, accurate imaging, and biopsy are essential to identify malignancy suitable for focal HIFU.

References

1. Chade DC, Shariat SF, Cronin AM, Savage CJ, Karnes RJ, Blute ML, et al. Salvage radical prostatectomy for radiation-recurrent prostate cancer: a multi-institutional collaboration. Eur Urol. 2011;60(2):205–10.
2. Murat FJ, Poissonnier L, Rabilloud M, Belot A, Bouvier R, Rouviere O, et al. Mid-term results demonstrate salvage high-intensity focused ultrasound (HIFU) as an effective and acceptably morbid salvage treatment option for locally radiorecurrent prostate cancer. Eur Urol. 2009;55(3):640–7.
3. Crouzet S, Murat FJ, Pommier P, Poissonnier L, Pasticier G, Rouviere O, et al. Locally recur-rent prostate cancer after initial radiation therapy: early salvage high-intensity focused ultra-sound improves oncologic outcomes. Radiother Oncol. 2012;105(2):198–202.
4. Uddin Ahmed H, Cathcart P, Chalasani V, Williams A, McCartan N, Freeman A, et al. Whole-gland salvage high-intensity focused ultrasound therapy for localized prostate cancer recur-rence after external beam radiation therapy. Cancer. 2012;118(12):3071–8.
5. Mouraviev V, Spiess PE, Jones JS. Salvage cryoablation for locally recurrent prostate cancer following primary radiotherapy. Eur Urol. 2012;61(6):1204–11.

6. Ahmed HU, Cathcart P, McCartan N, Kirkham A, Allen C, Freeman A, et al. Focal salvage therapy for localized prostate cancer recurrence after external beam radiotherapy: a pilot study. Cancer. 2012;118(17):4148–55.
7. Baco E, Gelet A, Crouzet S, Rud E, Rouvière O, Tonoli-Catez H, et al. Hemi salvage high-intensity focused ultrasound (HIFU) in unilateral radiorecurrent prostate cancer: a prospective two-centre study. BJU Int. 2014;114(4):532–40.
8. Nguyen PL, D'Amico AV, Lee AK, Suh WW. Patient selection, cancer control, and complications after salvage local therapy for postradiation prostate-specific antigen failure: a systematic review of the literature. Cancer. 2007;110(7):1417–28.
9. Heidenreich A, Richter S, Thuer D, Pfister D. Prognostic parameters, complications, and oncologic and functional outcome of salvage radical prostatectomy for locally recurrent prostate cancer after 21st-century radiotherapy. Eur Urol. 2010;57(3):437–43.
10. Chaussy C, Thuroff S, Bergsdorf T. Local recurrence of prostate cancer after curative therapy. HIFU (Ablatherm) as a treatment option. Urologe A. 2006;45(10):1271–5.
11. Hayashi M, Shinmei S, Asano K. Transrectal high-intensity focused ultrasound for treatment for patients with biochemical failure after radical prostatectomy. Int J Urol. 2007;14(11):1048–50.
12. Chaussy CG, Thuroff SF. Robotic high-intensity focused ultrasound for prostate cancer: what have we learned in 15 years of clinical use? Curr Urol Rep. 2011;12(3):180–7.

Focal Cryotherapy and COLD Database

10

John F. Ward

Content

Thermal tolerance is a cell's ability to withstand the extremes of temperature. In order to survive, a cell must maintain the integrity of the cellular boarders and extracellular matrix, as well as the quaternary structure of cytosol components and cellular metabolism. Heating beyond the upper thermal tolerance is the most common premise for many tissue ablative modalities (HIFU, interstitial laser). However, cryoablation uniquely takes advantage of a tissue's inability to survive temperatures beyond the lower end of the thermal viability spectrum. Surpassing the thermal viability limits at one extreme or the other may have more significant biologic implications than just a difference in temperature. Tissue death at these two extremes involves a very different set of mechanisms and as such may illicit a very different response from the body, regionally and systemically, that could offer both therapeutic advantages and an alternate morbidity profile. This difference may ultimately provide a rationale for choosing one form of tissue ablation over another (cryoablation over HIFU, as an example). However, for now, much of the decision to work at one end or the other of the thermal viability spectrum is based upon equipment availability and the comfort level of the surgeon with the energy source. Even datum to suggest a difference in morbidity between energy sources when applied in a focally ablative manner to treat prostate cancer remains scarce. It thus behooves the surgeon interested in focally ablative techniques for prostate cancer to be familiar and competent in a variety of energy sources for tissue ablation.

J.F. Ward, MD, FACS
Department of Urology, The University of Texas, M. D. Anderson Cancer Center,
Houston, TX, USA
e-mail: jfward@mdanderson.org

© Springer International Publishing Switzerland 2015
S. Thüroff, C.G. Chaussy (eds.), *Focal Therapy of Prostate Cancer:*
An Emerging Strategy for Minimally Invasive, Staged Treatment,
DOI 10.1007/978-3-319-14160-2_10

The temperature for prostate cancer cells at which 100 % cell death occurs is −19.4 °C [1]. Irrespective of the imaging modality used for guidance (magnetic resonance imaging, computed tomography, or ultrasonography), the operator cannot visualize a lethal isotherm of −20 °C but instead can visualize only the leading edge of the ice ball, which is approximately 0.5 °C, the temperature at which mammalian tissue freezes. Tissue effects may not be lethal at this temperature, leaving the potential for viable tissue, both cancerous and benign, to persist within the frozen zone. Studies considering the distance from the visible isotherm to the invisible lethal isotherm (−20 °C) have demonstrated a logarithmic decline in temperature from 0.5 to −25 °C within 3 mm of the visible isotherm and to −40 °C within 6 mm of the visible isotherm [1–3]. Therefore, a cryosurgeon must extend the visualized ice ball beyond the cancerous region to encompass the tissue within the lethal temperature zone. An extension of the ice beyond the prostate capsule threatens critical structures, such as the external sphincter, anterior rectum, and even the bladder base.

Cryoablation morbidity has been greatly reduced as the precision of the energy deposition was improved. The earliest applications of cryosurgery to treat prostate cancer involved transurethral freezing of the prostate with an inability to position the cryoneedles precisely or to monitor the extent of freezing beyond the transrectal palpation of a cold prostate [4]. While the early years of cryotherapy mirrored the early years of prostate cancer therapy with the goal of destroying all prostate tissue, as the technology for delivering lethal ice evolved from large liquid-nitrogen-driven probes to smaller, direct access gas-driven cryoprobes (Figs. 10.1 and 10.2) that allow a more precise conformation of the destruction zone, the morbidity associated with even whole gland cryoablation was significantly reduced. This improved precision not only reduced injury to surrounding critical structures but also has opened the possibility of preserving even nonmalignant portions of the prostate gland itself, i.e., focal cryotherapy.

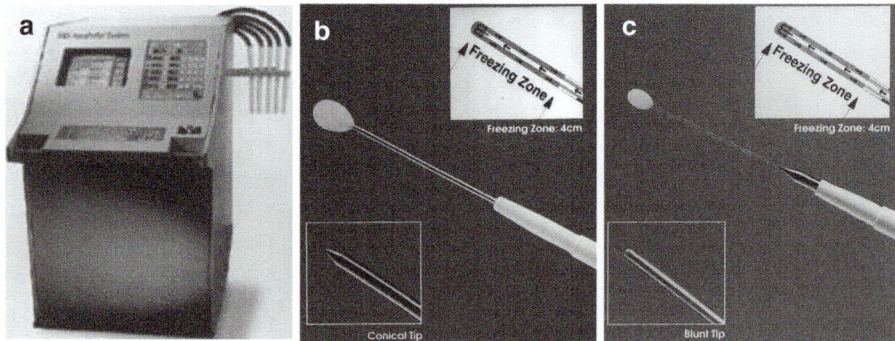

Fig. 10.1 CMS Accuprobe System 450 liquid nitrogen cryosurgical system. (**a**) The CMS Accuprobe System Model 450, a five-probe device; (**b**) flow schematic of a small-diameter cryoprobe capable of circulating liquid nitrogen within the tip's boiling chamber; (**c**, **d**) two of the various sizes and shapes of CMS cryoprobes: 3 mm × 4 cm × 18 cm probe with blunt tip (**c**) and 8 mm × 4 cm × 27 cm cryoprobe with conical tip (**d**)

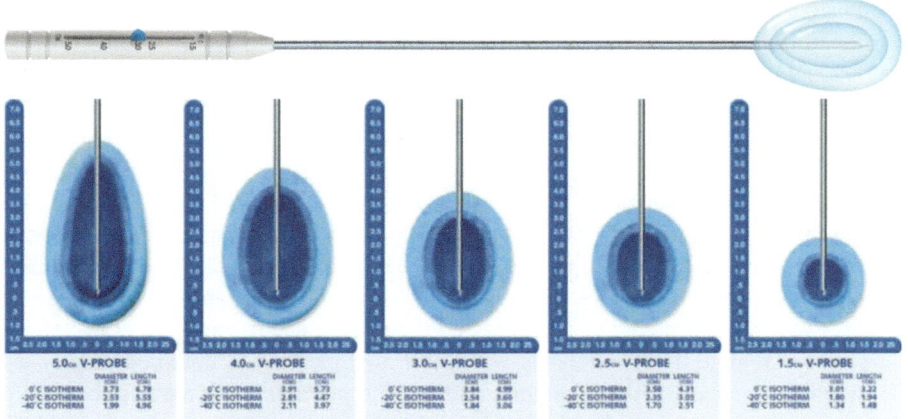

Fig. 10.2 Cryoprobe capable of producing ice of different lengths and shape to conform to the targeted area

In 2002, the current debate regarding focal therapy was ignited not de novo from within the urological community but from teams led by interventional radiologists. The first publication on prostate focal therapy all employed cryoablation as the thermally destructive energy source. Though the initial reports were both retrospective and lacked validated questionnaires to measure quality of life outcomes, they serve as truly ground breaking studies which catalyzed the current interest in the field regardless of the energy source deployed.

Onik and colleagues first reported on a series of 9 patients in 2002 [5] with a subsequent update to this series in 2008. From the updated series, 48 men submitted to hemispherical cryoablation with a minimum of 2 years of follow-up [6]. Patients were initially selected using transrectal Doppler biopsy and later by template mapping biopsy. Interestingly a majority of patients (52 %) were moderate or high risk according to D'Amico stratification. Using the original ASTRO definition of biochemical failure (3 successive increases in PSA), 94 % of the patients were free from biochemical recurrence, and no local recurrences were observed in the treated hemisphere. Of those men who were potent before hemiablation, 90 % (36/40) maintained potency "to the satisfaction of the patient." No incontinence was observed for any patients.

Bahn and colleagues contemporaneously yet separate from Onik reported in 2006 (mean follow-up of 70 months) on the outcomes of hemialative cryosurgery for 31 patients [7]. Patients treated in this series were selected for focal therapy based upon a standard 12-core, random prostate biopsy plus targeted biopsy of any suspicious regions of interest demonstrated with color Doppler. As with Onik, the original ASTRO definition of biochemical failure was used to define oncologic success. For this independent series, the outcomes were strikingly similar to the Onik series with 92.8 % (26/28) biochemically disease-free. Twenty-five patients underwent follow-up biopsy (again, random + Doppler guided) with 96.0 % (24/25) having no local evidence of disease. The single positive biopsy case was successfully salvaged with whole gland cryoablation. Potency, as determined with an administered non-validated questionnaire, was maintained by 88.9 % of patients (48.1 % (13/27) without and 40.7 % (11/27) with oral pharmaceutical assistance). Again, no incontinence was observed in this series.

While other small, single-surgeon, retrospective reports of focal therapy were published [8], the first major, multicenter publication of focal as it was being conducted in modern clinical practice emerged from the National Cryo On-Line Data (COLD) registry in 2012 [9]. This publication retrospectively reviewed the treatment of 5,853 men undergoing prostate cryoablation, of which 19.8 % ($n = 1,160$) underwent partial gland cryoablation. Similar to the Onik and Bahn series, this report was retrospective but incorporated the experience of multiple cryosurgeons trying to emulate those outcomes with their own patients in both community and academic practices. Unlike the Onik and Bahn reports, the volume and location of the treated prostate was determined by the treating cryosurgeon and not available for analysis. Similarly, the entry criteria were independently set by the treating cryosurgeon and not standardized across the 52 contributing sites.

This large, retrospective, data repository-driven report found a lower (75.7 %) freedom from biochemical recurrence-free rate (ASTRO definition) at 36 months than was observed in the earlier single-surgeon reports. Only 14.1 % of patients reported from the COLD registry treated with focal therapy underwent subsequent biopsy, assumed to be "for cause." Of those patients undergoing biopsy, 26.3 % (43/164) were positive for persistent disease. However, if one considers the entire cohort of patients and assumes that PSA can adequately predict the presence of persistent posttreatment cancer, the positive rate is 3.7 %, more consistent with the Onik/Bahn reports. Again, urinary continence (defined as use of 0 pads) was very high (98.4 %) though maintenance of spontaneous erections was not as successful with only 58.1 % who had spontaneous erections prior to organ preservation reporting return of erections to a baseline level. Morbidity of focal cryotherapy in this largest series, though much lower than following whole gland cryoablation, was not zero as in the earlier single-surgeon series; rather, prolonged urinary retention (>30 days) was reported in six (1.1 %) patients, and a single patient (0.1 %) did report a rectourethral fistula.

The first prospective study of focal therapy using cryoablation has now been reported by Barqawi and colleagues from the University of Colorado [10]. Unlike all prior reports of focal cryoablation where a treatment template incorporated the identified index lesion along with a wide swath of surrounding normal tissue (see Ward/Jones publication for the definitions of different organ-preserving focal templates [11]), in this prospective study, Barqawi et al. performed "targeted focal therapy" (TFT). In performing TFT, these investigators aimed to eradicate all clinically detected cancer foci rather than accepting the idea of the index lesion being the only clinically relevant tumor. In doing so, they have tried to more fully replicate the oncologic efficacy of radical therapy without the deleterious effects that can accompany whole gland treatment.

Low-risk disease (Gleason ≤ 7 (3+4) with less than 50 % positive core and 4 or fewer zones involved with cancer excluding the periurethral zone was identified in

62 men enrolled to this study between 2006 and 2009. All men underwent 3D mapping biopsy in order to qualify for treatment. The 3D mapping biopsy included placement of two gold fiducial markers for orientation and attainment of between four and eight cores from each of eight prostate zones yielding a total of 32–64 prostate biopsy cores. Targeted focal cryotherapy was performed between 8 and 12 weeks following mapping biopsy. A 17-gauge, gas-driven, variable length cryoprobe was positioned in all zones that showed at least one positive core on 3D mapping biopsy. Two freeze-thaw cycles to each zone were performed with a urethral warming catheter in place. At the conclusion of the treatment, the urethral warmer was exchanged for a Foley catheter, which remained in place for 1 week.

The primary end point of the study was 12-core TRUS-guided prostate biopsy within 12 months of treatment, rather than a repeat 3D mapping biopsy. Biochemical failure in this study was defined as postoperative PSA that equaled or exceeded preoperative PSA, due to the residual, untreated prostate tissue. AUA symptom scores and SHIM scores obtained preoperatively were compared to postoperative high and low scores obtained at any point postoperatively.

The median duration of this study at the time of report is 840 days. The 1-year repeat biopsy was negative in 50 of the 62 study subjects (81 %). The median PSA decrease over the study period was 3.0 ng/dl with 18 patients (29 %) experiencing a PSA rise over the course of their follow-up. Importantly, there was no significant change in the SHIM score following treatment, and the AUA symptom score declined 1.5 points ($p < 0.01$). No patients suffered urinary incontinence nor severe adverse events.

In conclusion, prostate cryotherapy has matured from its infancy when it was employed primarily to treat patients who failed primary radiation therapy and always in a radical fashion. With advances in the technology that has allowed more precise delivery of ablative energy to specified locations throughout the prostate, the third-generation technology has heralded the concept of precise targeting of cancer foci within the prostate gland in the hopes that this approach will ameliorate the morbidity associated with more radical treatments by preserving the non-diseased portions of the gland and the surrounding healthy tissue, including the urethral sphincter and the neurovascular bundles. While other energy sources are now available that can also be targeted to specific regions of the prostate, cryotherapy remains unique in its use of lethal, cold temperatures rather than heat. Differences in efficacy, morbidity, and even immunologic systemic responses between heating and cooling of prostate tissue have yet to be proven.

References

1. Kaouk JH, Aron M, Rewcastle JC, Gill IS. Cryotherapy: clinical end points and their experimental foundations. Urology. 2006;68:38–44.
2. Chosy SG, Nakada SY, Lee FT, Warner TF. Monitoring renal cryosurgery: predictors of tissue necrosis in swine. J Urol. 1998;159:1370–4.
3. Georgiades C, et al. Determination of the nonlethal margin inside the visible 'ice-ball' during percutaneous cryoablation of renal tissue. Cardiovasc Intervent Radiol. 2012. doi:10.1007/s00270-012-0470-5.

4. Gonder MJ, Soanes WA, SMITH V. Experimental prostate cryosurgery. Invest Urol. 1964;1:610–9.

5. Onik GM, Narayan P, Vaughan D, Dineen M, Brunelle R. Focal 'nerve-sparing' cryosurgery for treatment of primary prostate cancer: a new approach to preserving potency. Urology. 2002;60:109–14.

6. Onik GM, Vaughan D, Lotenfoe R, Dineen M, Brady J. The 'male lumpectomy': focal therapy for prostate cancer using cryoablation results in 48 patients with at least 2-year follow-up. Urol Oncol. 2008;26:500–5.

7. Bahn DK, et al. Focal prostate cryoablation: initial results show cancer control and potency preservation. J Endourol. 2006;20:688–92.

8. Ellis D, Manny TB, Rewcastle JC. Focal cryosurgery followed by penile rehabilitation as primary treatment for localized prostate cancer: initial results. Urology. 2007;70:9–15.

9. Ward JF, Jones JS. Focal cryotherapy for localized prostate cancer: a report from the national Cryo On-Line Database (COLD) Registry. BJU Int. 2012;109:1648–54.

10. Barqawi AB, et al. Targeted focal therapy in the management of organ-confined prostate cancer. J Urol. 2014;192:749–53. doi:10.1016/j.juro.2014.03.033. Epub 2014 Mar 15.

11. Ward JF, Jones JS. Classification system: organ preserving treatment for prostate cancer. Urology. 2010;75:1258–60.

Transrectal Prostate Cancer Ablation by Robotic High-Intensity Focused Ultrasound (HIFU) at 3 MHz: 18 Years Clinical Experiences

11

Stefan Thüroff and Christian G. Chaussy

Contents

S. Thüroff, MD (✉)
Department of Urology, Klinikum Harlaching,
Heinrich-Kröller-Str. 11, Munich D-81545, Germany
e-mail: sthueroff@mnet-mail.de

C.G. Chaussy, MD, FRCSEd (Hons)
University of Munich, Munich, Germany

Department of Urology, University of Regensburg, Regensburg, Germany

Keck School of Medicine, USC, Los Angeles, CA, USA
e-mail: cgchaussy@gmail.com

© Springer International Publishing Switzerland 2015
S. Thüroff, C.G. Chaussy (eds.), *Focal Therapy of Prostate Cancer:*
An Emerging Strategy for Minimally Invasive, Staged Treatment,
DOI 10.1007/978-3-319-14160-2_11

11.1   Introduction

Since the '30th it has been known experimentally that tissue can be destroyed from a distance by focused ultrasound [1]. However, clinical implementation of this principle was delayed due to the lack of a reliable technology. Today, computers, specific software, transrectal ultrasound devices, and MRI allow real-time therapy control and monitoring of HIFU treatment to achieve reproducible results.

Therefore, treatment with HIFU can now be extended to different surgical areas as a noninvasive method, which allows the coagulative destruction of tissue without an open surgical procedure. Increased experience and literature on HIFU has led to growing acceptance and use of transrectal HIFU for the treatment of prostate cancer worldwide. Clinical results with follow-up over 15 years have been published [2–6].

11.2   Physical Principle

The early use of HIFU for local tissue destruction was reported in 1944 by Lynn and Putman [7]. High-energy ultrasound parabolically focused on tissue leads to mechanical alteration of the cells and causes changes in biological structures (Fig. 11.1). During application of focused ultrasound, three different physical mechanisms can be observed: mechanical, thermal, and cavitation effects. Mechanical effects are induced by sudden pressure increase within the tissue by the HIFU beam being highly energetic. This energy input into the tissue induces formation of cavitation bubbles within the tissue. This mechanical cavitation effect damages cell membranes.

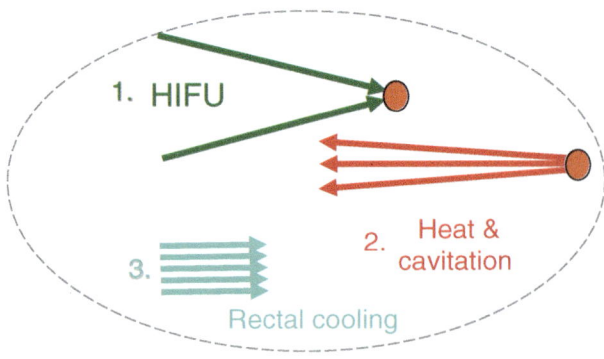

Fig. 11.1 Physical principle of focused energy application

Fig. 11.2 Multiple lesion application= volume coagulation

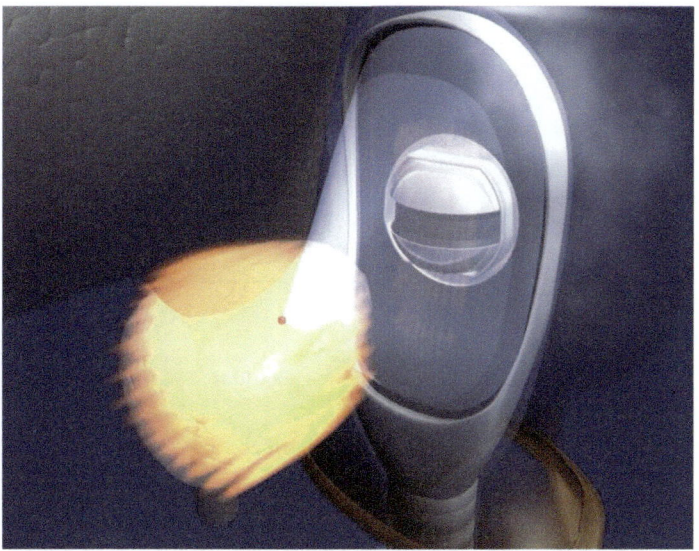

A thermal effect is caused by the absorption of ultrasonic energy within the tissue. The temperature increase in tissues depends on the absorption coefficient of the tissue and the size, shape, and temperature sensitivity of the heated area. Biological changes caused by the heating depend on the temperature level and duration of exposure. A "thermal dose," which exceeds a certain threshold, causes tissue coagulation and leads to irreversible tissue damage [8]. High-intensity focused ultrasound generates a very high intensity in the focal area, causes high temperatures within a few seconds (85 °C), and destroys the tissue in a circumscribed area while surrounding areas remain unharmed. The defined small tissue volume, which is destroyed by one single ultrasonic beam, is a "primary" lesion. In order to coagulate larger areas, multiple lesions have to be added in a certain algorithm (Fig. 11.2). This can be achieved by motorized computer-controlled movement of the energy source or by an electronically "phased array" [8–13].

11.3   Technology

Important HIFU setting parameters are as follows:

- Therapeutic and diagnostic ultrasound frequency (3/7.5 MHz)
- Acoustic high intensity (40–50 W)
- Duration of HIFU application (shot/lesion time)
- Intervals between HIFU pulses (delay time)
- Lateral shift between elementary lesions (rotation angle)
- Longitudinal displacement of applicator (slice thickness 1.7 mm)
- Penetration depth (focal point dependent on the applicator design/device)

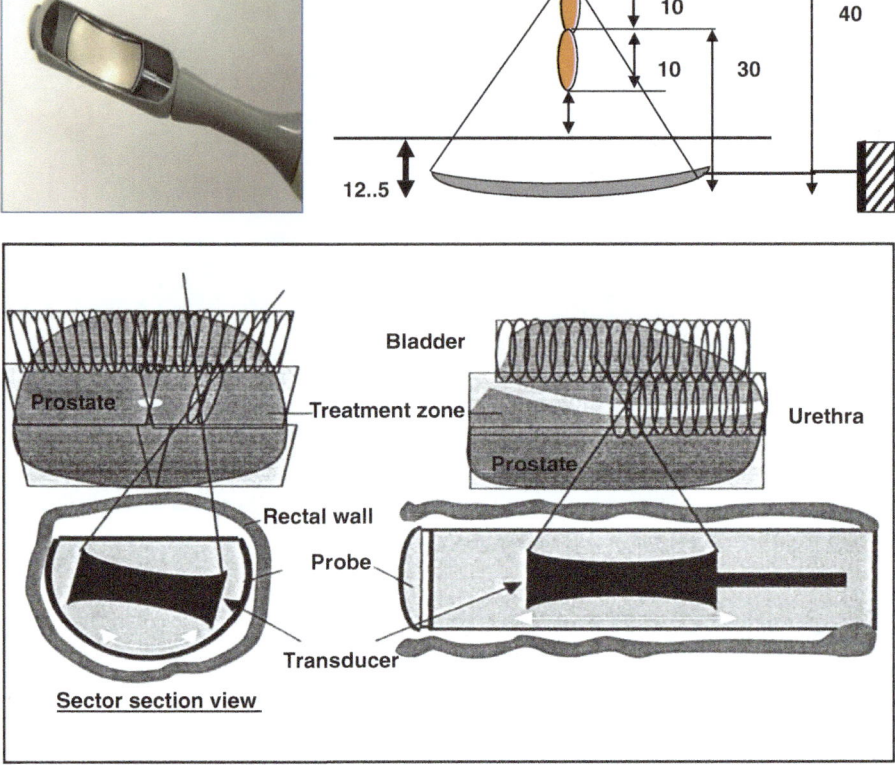

Fig. 11.3 Sonablate® applicator and lesion formation principle

These technical parameters are essential in the assembly of a HIFU system for specific tissue and a dedicated application. Besides this, difficult technical decisions concern the selection and design of the piezoelectric energy applicator, the imaging system, the intraoperative target and safety features, the target localization during treatment (TRUS or MRI), and the therapy controls (robotic and/or visually guided). The therapeutic ultrasonic energy transducer is characterized mainly by the operating frequency and the geometric and physical design (Fig. 11.3a, b).

Piezoelectric systems can be operated with sufficient energy density, reproducibility, and long-term stability in accordance with the requirements of the therapy which allow the production of geometric shapes in order to adapt them to the different anatomical needs [11]. Current standard urological applications use "single-focus" HIFU transducers which are adjustable mechanical movements or combinations out of mechanical and phased array applicators (Fig. 11.4 and 11.5).

To find the ultrasound parameters that are required for the treatment of prostatic tissue, in vitro and in vivo experiments have been performed for more than a decade, as computer simulation systems have been developed [14]. MRI is one technique to assess the effectiveness of HIFU treatment and can perform

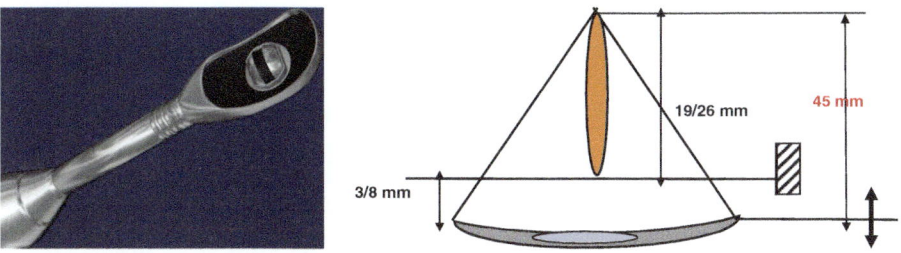

Fig. 11.4 Ablatherm® applicator and lesion formation principle

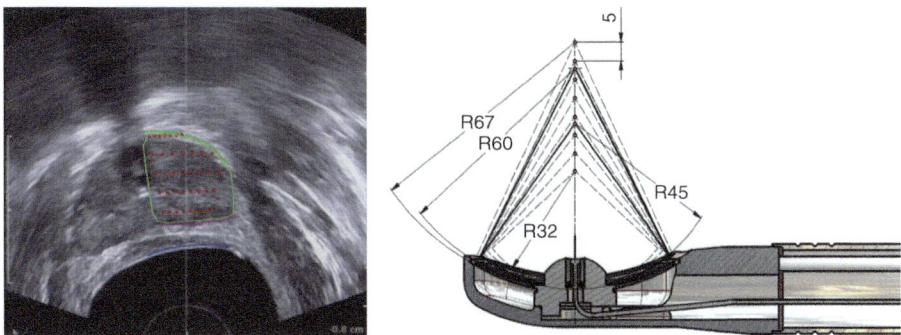

Fig. 11.5 Focal.One® applicator and lesion formation principle

real-time temperature measurements. MRI is used in extracorporeal HIFU treatments rather than transrectal approach for localization and monitoring effectiveness [15] and allows the measurement of temperature changes during HIFU treatment [16]. Studies have used magnetic resonance elastography (MRE) to investigate the effects of temperature-induced tissue ablation by measuring the mechanical changes of the lesion [17].

> It remains unclear whether instant elastography changes can be correlated to intermittent edema-induced reduced blood flow or whether they reflect irreversible tissue coagulation at a cellular level.

HIFU-induced lesions are temporarily seen as TRUS hyperdense areas [18]. This optical effect disappears after 10 min. However, the real extent of a primary lesion cannot be defined precisely, because effects such as HIFU reflection (prostatic capsule, calcifications, catheters), absorption (untreated or pretreated tissue), and cooling (blood vessels, intraprostatic TUR cavity liquid) are individually different. Further characterization techniques based on ultrasound, contrast-enhanced Doppler [19], or different techniques to the acoustic behavior of tissues have been proposed to determine the extent of HIFU-induced lesions.

During 18 years of clinical experience with HIFU in prostate cancer, it has been proven that transrectal ultrasound is safe for reproducible clinical application even without sophisticated "real-time" temperature measurement. Still a "real-time" technology, compensating the above mentioned individual tissue effects would be favorable and optimize tissue ablation safety and efficacy.

11.4   Experimental Preclinical History

Destruction of tissue with HIFU has been studied in various experimental tumor models. To study the HIFU effect in vivo, experiments were performed on mouse glioma [20], hamster medulloblastoma [21], and rat Morris hepatoma [22, 23]. DUNNING R3327 and AT2 and AT6 carcinomas with high metastatic potential [24, 25], implanted in rats, were studied as models of prostate cancer.

In vitro [26, 27], ex vivo [26, 28], and in vivo [16, 27, 29] experiments were also performed to study the treatment possibilities with HIFU for kidney tumors. These animal studies provided evidence that cancerous tissue can be destroyed with HIFU without inducing metastasis [25]. Transrectal HIFU for treatment of the prostate was confirmed in experimental canine models [30, 31].

11.5   Transrectal HIFU Devices

After attempts to treat BPH with HIFU proved unsuccessful [32–34], transrectal HIFU as treatment of prostate cancer has found its way into routine clinical practice. Within the last decade, solely Ablatherm has treated more than 35,000 patients worldwide for PCa with HIFU®.

Transrectal HIFU does not de-obstruct BPH but induces instant necrosis, and on long terms tissue shrinkage. It induces obstruction by necrotic and scar tissue.

Two devices for the transrectal approach have been designed and are routinely manufactured and marketed out of the United States for the treatment of prostate cancer.

Clinical significant results are available from Sonablate® (Focus Surgery Inc., Indianapolis) [6, 10, 32, 57] and Ablatherm® (EDAP TMS SA, Vaulx-en-Velin, France) [2–5] (Figs. 11.6 and 11.7). Prostate cancer ablation by HIFU has been studied as well in a European Ablatherm® multicenter study as in other prospective studies and described in detail [35, 36]. The authors reported separately

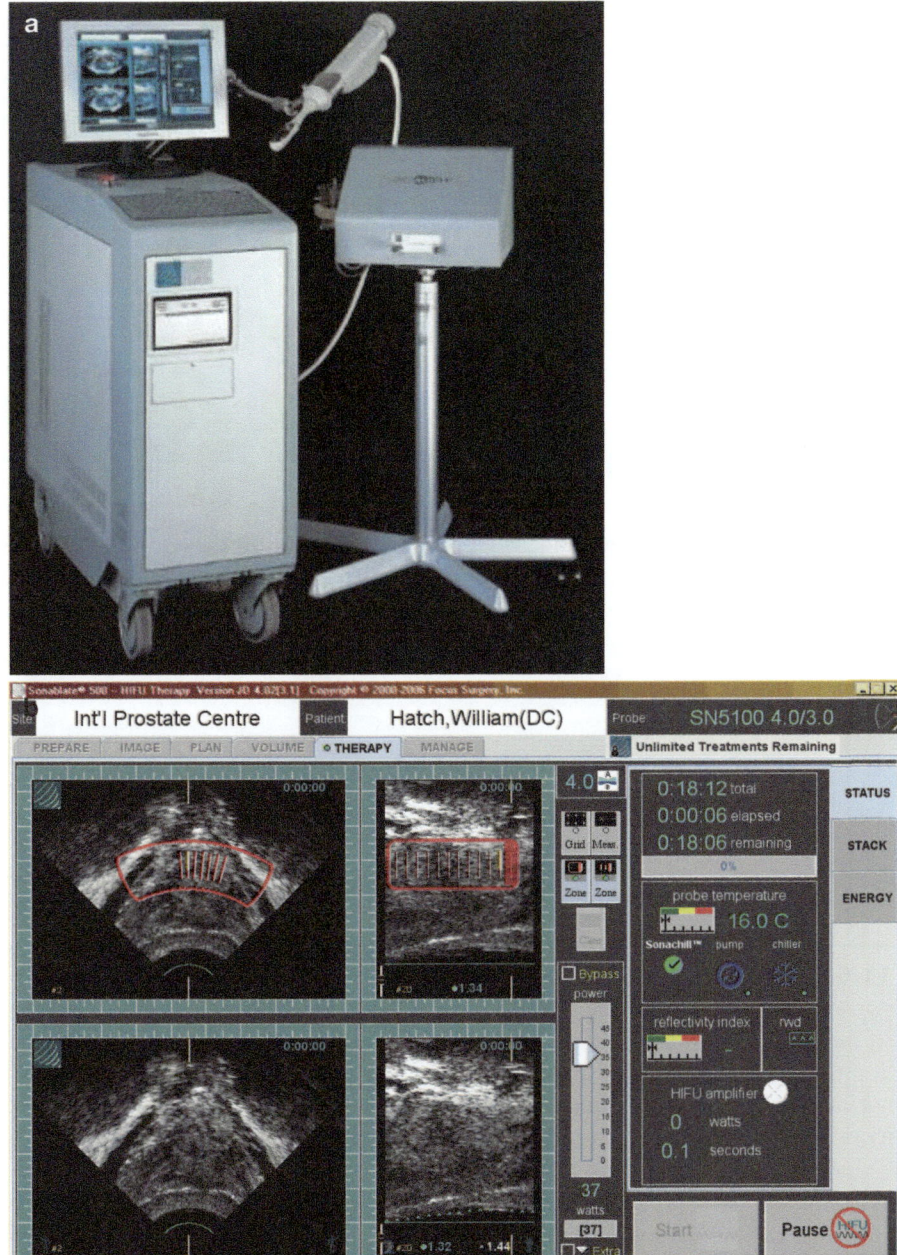

Fig. 11.6 Sonablate® 500. (**a**) Device. (**b**) Operators interface/monitor. (**c**) Patient's therapy position

Fig. 11.6 (continued)

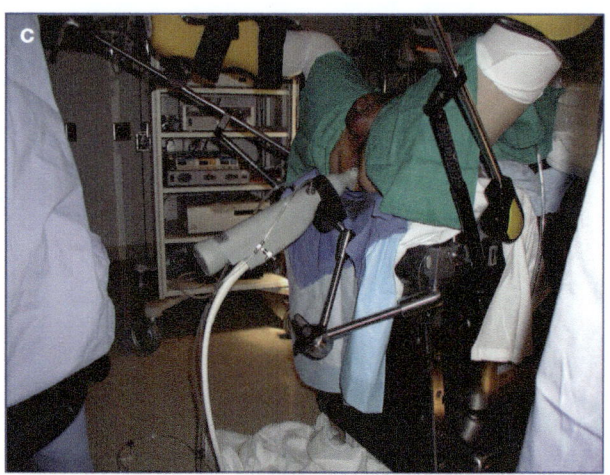

about their experiences in defined patient groups and established – on the basis of these results – standardized procedures and protocols for patient management.

> For both devices, FDA approval is pending; requested studies have been already terminated but not yet published. The authors worked for 18 years with Ablatherm® only, their clinical and published experience is related to this specific technology. Clinical results cannot be simply pooled to other HIFU technologies.

11.6   Indications and Contraindications for Ablatherm®

At the beginning of the first clinical studies of our Munich group 1996, the indication for HIFU was restricted to patients with localized prostate cancer who were not candidates for surgery due to their age, general health status, and/or comorbidity or patients who decided definitively against radiation or radical prostatectomy.

Indications and application mode have been expanded over the following years – based on clinical experience of this first study. These expanded indications included partial and focal therapy in low-risk tumors, incidental prostate cancer after TUR, and salvage therapy in recurrent prostate cancer after radical prostatectomy, radiotherapy, and previous HIFU.

Besides the indications in localized PCa, pilot studies showed that adjuvant non-invasive cytoreduction by HIFU in locally advanced prostate cancer, even in minimal metastatic stages and for progressive castration-resistant prostate cancer (CrPCa), could achieve promising results.

Contraindications for transrectal HIFU are rare: missing or small rectum; a damaged, tumor-infiltrated or infected rectal wall caused by previous prostatic/rectal therapies; or severe Latex allergy (balloon).

11.7   TURP Before HIFU

TURP prior to HIFU allows the instant removal of any reflecting, deviating, or absorbing calcifications, abscesses, intravesical middle lobes, and adenomas, and it should prevent later infravesical obstruction.

> As it is well accepted that a total prostate volume can be downsized by 30 % within 3 months by androgen deprivation therapy (ADT), this could not substitute TURP before HIFU because of the necessity of removal of intraprostatic calcifications, intravesical middle lobes, intraprostatic abscesses, and bigger adenomas.

The generation of an intraprostatic cavity by TUR and its subsequent intratherapeutic compression by the rectal balloon increase the accessibility of the HIFU waves to the remaining gland (Fig. 11.7), fix the residual prostate behind the symphysis bone, and prevent movement artifacts during HIFU application [37, 38].

> Increase of invasiveness by neoadjuvant TURP is compensated by the beneficial effects in regard to higher efficacy and lower side effects as well as it expands the indication range for HIFU.

The beneficial effect of a combination of TUR and HIFU was demonstrated in a series of 271 patients with prostate cancer and an initial PSA of <15 ng/ml.

Ninety-six of 271 patients received HIFU monotherapy, while 175 were treated with combination therapy. The mean resection weight was 15.7 g (2–110 g), median 12.5 g. The mean follow-up time in the monotherapy group was 18.7 ± 12.1 months and for the combination therapy group was 10.9 ± 6.2 months. The histological results in both groups were similar after treatment, with negative biopsies in 87.7 % versus 81.6 %. The median PSA Nadir was <0.1 ng/ml in both groups. The monotherapy group required a suprapubic catheter for 40 days, while in the combination group it was removed after 7 days. With this study, the benefits of a combination therapy could be demonstrated [36].

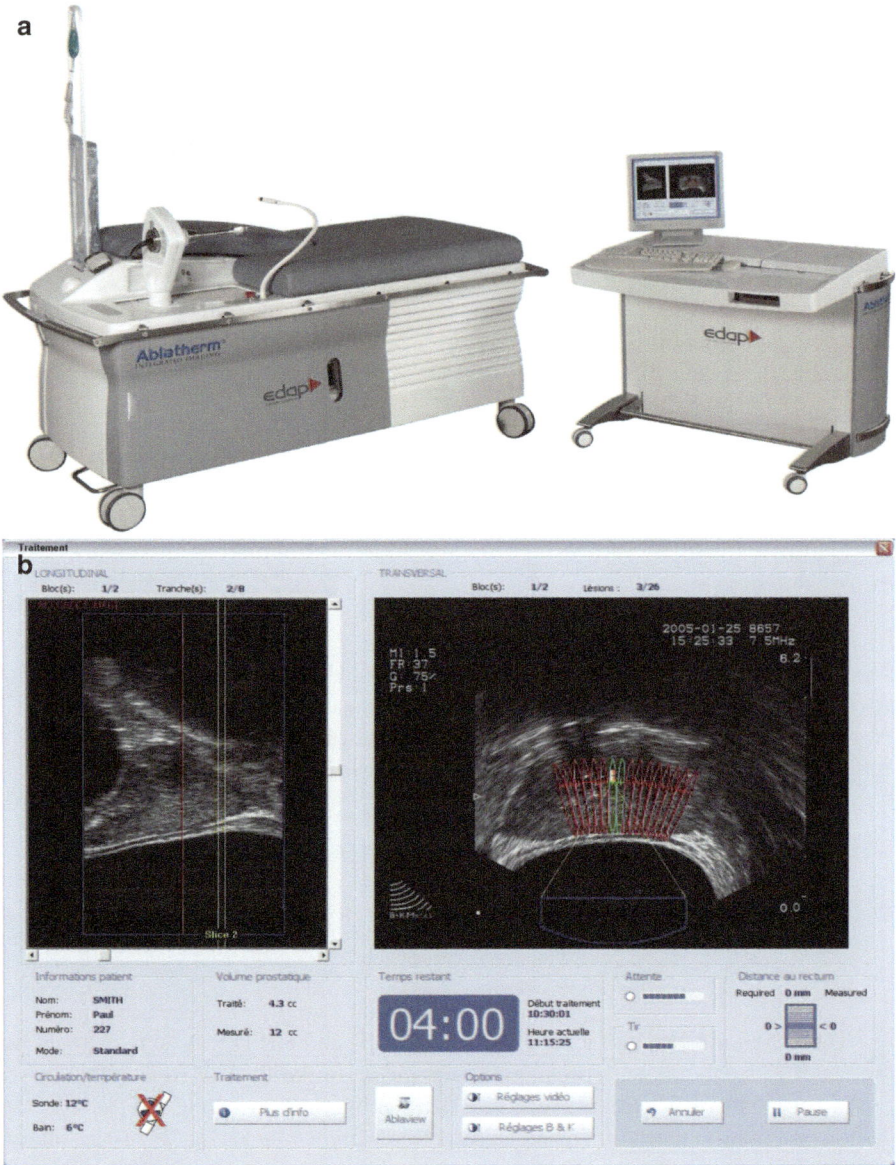

Fig. 11.7 Ablatherm® integrated imaging. (**a**) Device. (**b**) Operators interface/monitor. (**c**) Patient's therapy position

Fig. 11.7 (continued)

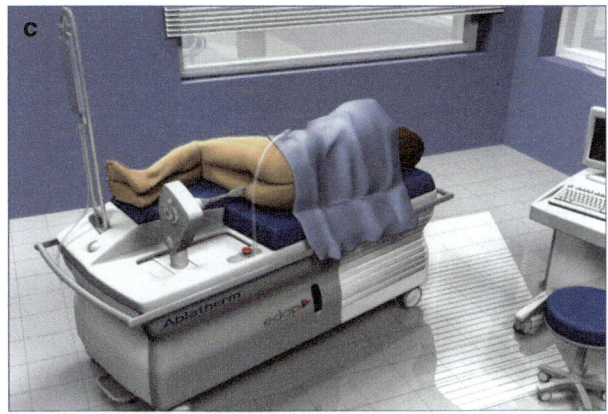

11.8 HIFU Effect on Prostate Tissue

Despite the fact that bioptic controls have a low significance in relation to their random character, they can show and prove the instant intraprostatic ablative effect of the HIFU procedure and the long-term replacement of prostatic by fibrotic tissue.

In a clinical study, in which a partial HIFU treatment was performed 1–2 weeks before radical prostatectomy, the instant efficacy of HIFU was histologically confirmed after complete prostate removal. HIFU had been applied to the sites where positive tissue biopsies had been found. Histological examination of the samples showed a sharp demarcation between the HIFU-treated and untreated areas, while in the treated areas complete necrosis was found [39].

The extent of tissue damage caused by HIFU can be determined by gadolinium-enhanced MRI. The treated area appears as a hypodense zone surrounded by a strong 3–8 mm peripheral rim. This corresponds to histopathological findings characterized by a core of coagulation necrosis surrounded by a peripheral zone of inflammation.

> Immunological research hypothesis judges this "heat deactivated but not totally ablated cancer tissue" (microscopically alive but in immune histological staining dead cells) as individual trigger for immunitary response – in sense of "cancer vaccination."

The treatment-induced MRI changes usually disappear within 3–5 months and the HIFU-induced contraction of the tissue results after about 6 months in small prostates of approximately 5–7 cc [40].

> This strong fibrotic shrinkage process can induce side effects as formation of intraprostatic or bladder neck stenosis in up to 15 % within the first 12 months.

This occurs specifically after "radical" HIFU (TUR and complete HIFU) shows prevalence in smaller glands and is combined in most cases with perfect oncological outcome (PSA = "0").

11.9   HIFU in Primary, Localized Prostate Cancer (T1–2)

The prognosis of treatment outcome in PCa patients treated with radical prostatectomy is – beside PSA Nadir and PSA velocity after Nadir – based on pathological features such as tumor grade, stage, and margin status.

Due to the absence of histological specimens following HIFU, it is necessary to focus on PSA Nadir as a predictor of clinical failure. It has been evaluated and shown to be the strongest surrogate factor of treatment failure [41] in HIFU as well.

In addition, the PSA Nadir was strongly associated with both preoperative PSA level and residual prostate volume. PSA Nadir effects in patients with a longer follow-up have been reported by Ganzer et al. [42].

It was shown that the PSA Nadir after HIFU correlated highly significantly with treatment failure and disease-free survival rate (DFSR). Treatment failure rates during follow-up were 4.5, 30.4, and 100 %, respectively, for three different PSA Nadir groups ($P < 0.001$). The actuarial disease-free survival rates at 5 years were 95, 55, and 0 %, respectively ($P < 0.001$).

These findings suggest that oncological outcome is improved if a PSA Nadir of ≤ 0.2 ng/ml (without additional ADT) is reached after 3 months.

In a series of 120 patients with localized prostate cancer and PSA values of <10 ng/ml, cancer-free survival rates were examined. These patients were not suitable for radical prostatectomy and had a life expectancy of 10 years [2]. The calculated cancer-free 5-year survival rate for the average patient population was 76.9 %; this was significantly increased to 85.4 % in highly differentiated tumors (Gleason score 2–6) compared to 61.3 % in low-differentiated tumors (Gleason score 7–10). There was no significant difference in survival rates calculated in terms of prostate volume or the number of positive biopsies. Nadir PSA is seen as the prognostic factor with a theoretical 5-year survival rate of 86 % in patients with a Nadir PSA <0.5 ng/ml [43, 44].

An early European Ablatherm® multicenter study reported short-term results of 402 patients with localized prostate cancer (T1–2/N0-x/M0) between 1995 and 1999, 1 year after HIFU treatment [35]. 87.2 % of control biopsies were negative. Classified – according to the prognostic risk – in the group with low risk (Gleason <7), 92.1 % were negative, in the medium-risk group (Gleason 7) 86.4 %, and in the high-risk group (Gleason > 7) 82.1 %. PSA Nadir was found in average 2–3 months after HIFU treatment. The prostate volume in relation to the completeness of the HIFU treatment significantly influenced PSA after treatment. PSA remained stable after treatment during the mean follow-up of 407 days.

Blana et al. reported a study of 140 patients with localized prostate cancer [45]. These patients had a baseline PSA value of ≤15 ng/ml and a Gleason score of ≤7. TRUS biopsies 6 months following HIFU treatment were negative in 93.4 % of patients. The mean PSA Nadir was 0.07 ng/ml and the PSA value remained during a mean observation period of 22 months at 0.16 ng/ml. In 77 % and 69 % respectively, there was no biochemical relapse after 5 and 7 years, respectively. Although a satisfactory "cure" rate in patients with low- and medium-risk disease has been observed with HIFU as monotherapy, combination therapy should be considered for patients with high-risk disease. In this study, no severe incontinence (grade II–III) could be found. Because of a urinary obstruction 12 % of the patients needed a transurethral resection during the follow-up period. In 47.3 % of patients, potency could be maintained and there were no reports of significant changes in International Prostate Symptom Scores (IPSS). The 5-year survival rates of this study correspond to the large series of standard treatments of localized prostate cancer [46–51], [82].

> Our long-term results [1] in T1–2 PCa show in a cohort of 704 patients with a maximum follow-up of 14 years (median follow-up 5.5 years) that at 10 years 2/3rd of the patients are biochemically disease-free (Phoenix criteria) and that ¾ did not need another salvage therapy.

11.10 HIFU in Incidental PCa

Up to 8 % of patients who undergo TURP/adenectomy for BPH show unexpected PCa in histology [52]. Based on this experience we performed a prospective monocentric pilot study, treated and followed 78 patients since 2000, and could prove that the three most important oncological success criteria after HIFU are "PSA Nadir" of 0.07 ng/ml, "PSA velocity" in a 10-year follow-up of 0.01 ng/ml/year, and "no further salvage therapy" in combination with minimal side effect rate, proved perfect oncological outcome [53].

> Even if TUR-detected tumor volume, initial PSA, and Gleason score staged a "low-risk tumor," some patients opt out of psychological reasons for a noninvasive single-session HIFU therapy rather than "wait and see," "watchful waiting," or even radical surgical or radiation approach. HIFU is the only therapy profiting out of the previous TUR!

11.11 Training and Costs

Nowadays, the acceptance of a new cancer therapy is influenced not only by its onco-logical efficacy or side effects but also very much by its costs and reimbursement issues. Local costs have to be analyzed by the user and accepted by the reimbursing authority and the patient. Direct and indirect costs have to be considered, and costs have to be compared to alternative therapies already existing [55]. Cost reduction is, that HIFU by Ablatherm® is a mobile system: it needs neither installation nor specific external conditions. As a patient bed, it passes normal doors and elevators. It is a "roll-in-roll-off" or "plug-and-play" device, which can be set up in start conditions within 15 min after entering a room – important for mobile use and OR occupation.

Just a 16 A electric plug and anesthesia support are needed to perform therapy; no specific sterile operation room needs to be occupied.

> HIFU or "TUR and HIFU" is a "one-man show": a urologist and an anesthe-siologist are necessary during this 2.5 h treatment, so it is staff saving (less staff for a complex robotic surgery is not possible).

Training of new users is standardized since >10 years [83–86].

There is "on-site backup" by experienced coach or application specialist until the new user feels comfortable, mostly after about ten treatments. As perioperative side effects are rare and hospitalization is short, the additional costs are homogeneous and easy to calculate.

> While most other treatment options for localized prostate cancer (e.g., sur-gery, radiation, cryotherapy, or brachytherapy) cannot be repeated in cases of local PCa recurrence, HIFU for PCa can be repeated safely (not after previous radiation!) and shows to be even more effective the second time [54].

11.12 Side Effects After Primary, Localized HIFU

Today's observed side effects after HIFU for prostate cancer are mainly intermedi-ate voiding dysfunction and retention caused by edema, necrosis, or bladder outlet obstruction at 6–12 months [2–4, 6].

Severe side effects such as rectourethral fistula [56–58], grade II–III urinary incon-tinence, or permanent bladder outlet obstruction occurred and referred in most cases on the prototype devices without cooling, without real-time visualization, and without robotic autofocus applicator adjustment. Prevalence of side effects was as in therapeu-tic salvage situations (i.e., locally recurrent PCa after surgery and radiation).

It is important to mention that side effects typically occur within the first months and decrease up to maximum of one year. Later primary onset of side effects is unknown.

In none of our treatments have been occurred any intra- or perioperative severe side effects: (no emergency surgery, no blood transfusions, no intensive care, no thrombosis or pulmonary embolism) occurred. This shows the low invasiveness of the therapy.

Finally, there is no general "Gleason shift" to more aggressive stages in recurrent PCa after HIFU seen, as it typically happens after ADT or radiation therapy [59].

Recurrent PCa after HIFU has a smaller volume (<10 cc) than before and can be retreated by HIFU without increased morbidity, if there has not been previous radiation therapy [54].

To reduce postoperative urethral catheter time and postoperative morbidity (sludging, obstruction, infection), prospective studies were undertaken to observe the effect of a combination therapy (HIFU and TUR). In a pilot study in 30 patients with localized prostate cancer, a one-stage (in same anesthesia) combination therapy with TUR and HIFU was performed. Mean treatment duration was 2:48 h. The transurethral catheter time was 2 days and the mean hospitalization 3 days. After 6 months, control biopsies were negative in 80 % of patients, and the median PSA was 0.9 ng/ml. Mean Post-treatment International Prostate Symptom Score (PIPSS) was 6.7, compared with a pretreatment score of 7.5. Potency was preserved in 73 % of patients who had reported no erectile dysfunction before treatment [35].

Today's rate of adverse events among patients with primary – not salvage – therapy is low in regard to stress incontinence: grade I° is observed in 4–6 % of patients and grade II in 2 %, but secondary infravesical obstruction is seen in up to 25 %. Severe incontinence (grade III) and urethra–rectal fistulae are rare (<1 %) since the introduction of robotic rectal HIFU integrating with real-time visualization (since 2005) (Figs. 11.4 and 11.7a).

Preservation of erectile function is directly dependent on the position of the primary lesion in relation to the neurovascular bundle (complete, partial, or focal treatment) (Figs. 11.8 and 11.9b). Although sparing the contralateral side for neurovascular preservation can improve potency, it results in a higher local failure and consequent HIFU retreatment rate [49–52].

11.13   Salvage Prostatectomy After HIFU

Before introduction of the combination therapy (TUR + HIFU) we performed seven radical prostatectomies after HIFU between 1996 and 2000. This was due to initially incomplete HIFU treatments of larger-size prostates. As the application of

HIFU causes severe fibrotic adhesions between the rectum and Denovillier's fascia, radical prostatectomy after HIFU is surgically more demanding; however, in our experience it was not associated with higher morbidity compared to a standard prostatectomy, and it was easier than prostatectomy after radiation therapy.

Since the introduction of "TUR before HIFU," radical prostatectomy is rare and difficult, because now the prostate volume is small and the resected bladder neck fibrotic: so HIFU should not be misunderstood by the patient as a "trial and error" procedure before a potential radical surgery, and a patient has to be informed about this.

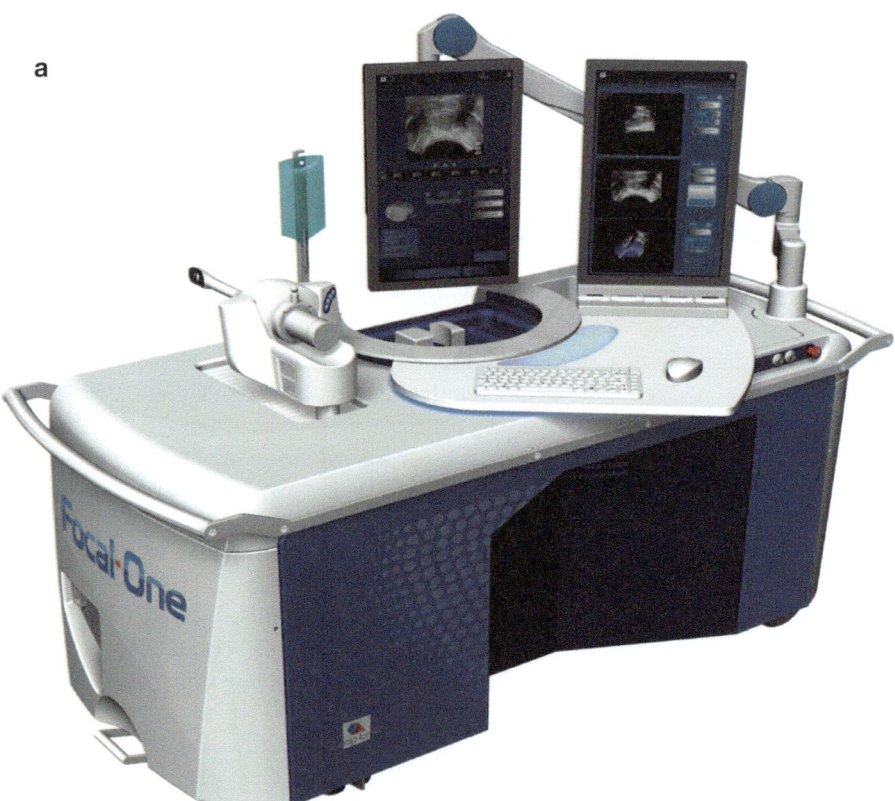

Fig. 11.8 Focal.One®. (**a**) Device. (**b**) Operators interface/monitor. (**c**) Patient's therapy position

Fig. 11.8 (continued)

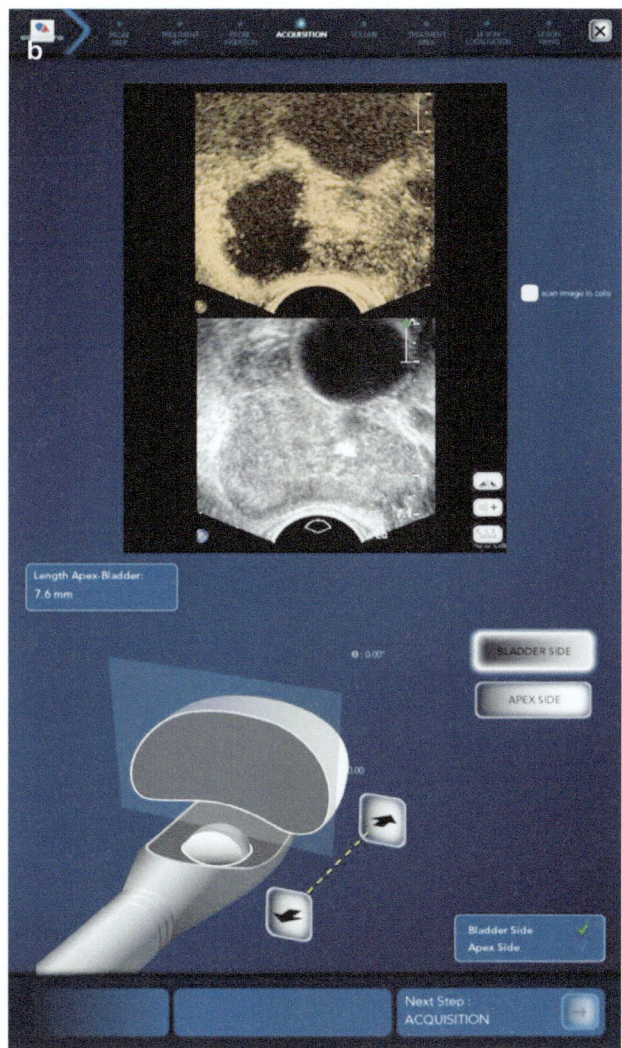

c

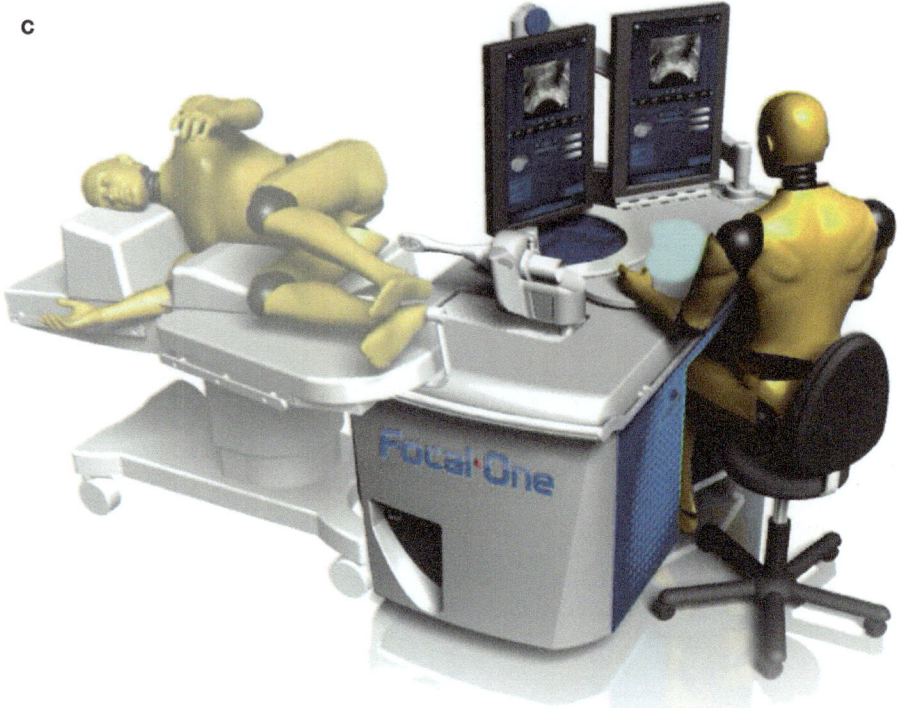

Fig. 11.8 (continued)

a

b

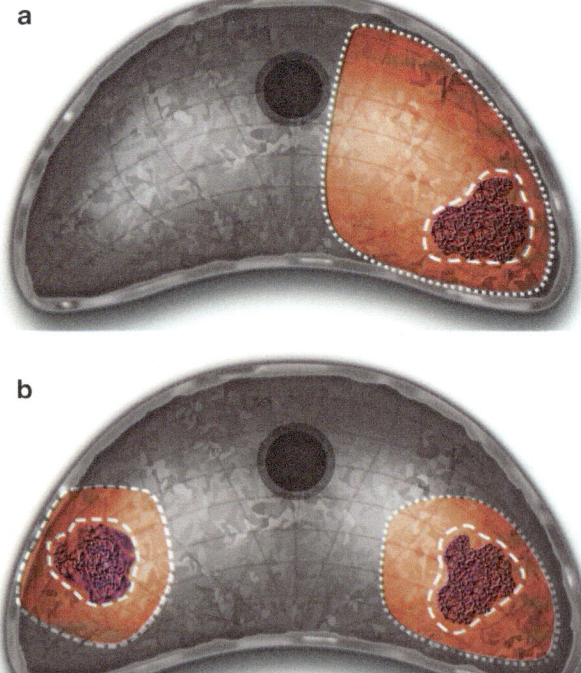

Fig. 11.9 Focal Prostata
cancer. (**a**) Monofocal –
hemiablation. (**b**)
Mulitfocal – safety
margin ablation

11.14 Salvage HIFU After Brachytherapy

Limited experience exists with HIFU following brachytherapy, but it appears that this approach is not associated with a significant increase in complications compared to primary HIFU [61]. It is definitively advisable to monitor the position of the seeds precisely before HIFU (TRUS/MR).

> There should be no seeds outside the prostate capsule, especially not between the rectum and the prostate. In these areas, they would interfere with the direct entry path of the ultrasound. Intraprostatic seeds seem not to disturb.

11.15 Salvage HIFU After Radical Prostatectomy

Therapeutic options for local recurrence following radical prostatectomy are limited and typically it is radiation therapy. Even here, failure rate is 67 % at 4 years (CaPsure database). HIFU offers an additional treatment option when local recurrence can be identified through transrectal ultrasound and verified by biopsies. After treatment with HIFU, the treated areas showed negative biopsies in 77 %. The PSA Nadir averaged 0.2 ng/ml and 66 % of the patients achieved PSA Nadir values <0.5 ng/ml. During follow-up of 5 years, 91 % of the patients showed no biochemical progress [62, 63].

> Personal experience showed that best – even curative – results could be achieved when patients had a recurrent PSA < 1 n/ml, related to a small and defined tumor volume. In cases with bigger local recurrent tumors and higher PSA levels, salvage HIFU after surgery served to stop the regrowth of residual cancer tissue after a locally debulking TUR.

> The major side effect after this salvage procedure was urinary stress incontinence. We experienced that patients without post-surgery incontinence did better than patients with a longer incontinence history (probably their continence was caused by recurrent tumor growth) [62, 63].

11.16 Salvage HIFU After Radiation Therapy

HIFU treatments have been performed as salvage therapy following external radiotherapy failures. A. Gelet reported results of 71 patients [64]. All patients were diagnosed with a biochemical recurrence and local disease confirmed by biopsies.

In one third of patients, androgen deprivation was employed either as a measure to auxiliary radiotherapy or early biochemical relapse, prior to HIFU treatment. During follow-up after HIFU, 80 % of treated patients showed negative biopsies (median follow-up period of 14.8, 6–86 months). The median PSA Nadir was 0.2 ng/ml. In patients with HIFU as salvage therapy after external radiotherapy, a significantly higher rate of side effects is observed, compared with patients who undergo primary HIFU therapy. Nevertheless, there is a favorable risk–benefit ratio after HIFU treatment as compared to the alternatives [64–68], [81].

> HIFU as therapeutic treatment option for recurrent prostate cancer is salvage therapy option is included in most European guidelines (France, Italy, Germany): if it works there why shouldn't it be even more effective in primary indications as well?

11.17 Cytoreductive Supportive HIFU in Advanced PCa

Pilot study results for the palliative treatment of advanced prostate cancer with HIFU show promising results in terms of reduction in local morbidity (rectal compression, infravesical obstruction, hydronephrosis, hematuria, pelvic pain syndromes) as well as in PSA reduction and salvage treatment-free survival. Published data in monocentric group ($n = 143$) in T3 and CrPCa cases with follow-up of 10 years show a post-HIFU low PSA velocities of 0.17 ng/ml/year in favorable T3 disease (PSAi < 20 ng/ml and without additional hormone ablation). Local tumor ablation with HIFU also resulted in a PSA reduction of 83 % in HRPCa cases. There was also evidence of a synergistic effect in hormone ablative therapies, with delays seen in the onset of hormone resistance [60].

11.18 Cytoreductive HIFU in Castration-Resistant PCa (CrPCA)

Castration resistance after long-term ADT occurs in most cases after years, in high-Gleason tumors faster than in low-Gleason tumors. As ADT is not curative but only palliative, it should not be started too early. Therapeutic options in ADT-resistant progressive PCa are rare and poor. We performed a pilot study to evaluate HIFU efficacy in this specific patient group and could show a 84 % PSA decrease and delay of disease (return of PSA to level at inclusion) of years [60]

11.19 Immunological Induction by HIFU?

Recent progress has been made in developing an effective immune strategy for treating prostate cancer. A number of immunotherapy regimens are being studied including immune-modulating cytokines/effectors, peptide and cellular immunization, viral vaccines, dendritic cell vaccines, and antibody therapies. Immune-modulating agents, such as granulocyte–macrophage colony-stimulating factor (GM-CSF), Flt3 ligand, and IL-2, have been used to stimulate the immune system to generate an antitumor response against prostate cancer.

Several recent studies have looked at the potential of HIFU to initiate an immune response. Especially Asian scientists published about the effect of HIFU on systemic antitumor immunity, particularly T-lymphocyte-mediated immunity in cancer patients.

They investigated whether the tumor antigens expressed on breast cancer cells may be preserved after HIFU treatment. Primary tumors in 23 patients with biopsy-proven breast cancer were treated with HIFU, than submitted to modified radical mastectomy. Breast cancer specimens were then stained for a variety of cellular molecules, including tumor antigens and heat-shock protein 70 (HSP-70).

A number of tumor antigens were identified, and these could provide a potential antigen source to stimulate antitumor immune response.

It has been suggested that endogenous signals from HIFU-damaged tumor cells may trigger the activation of dendritic cells and that this may play a critical role in a HIFU-elicited antitumor immune response.

Status of tumor-infiltrating lymphocytes (TILs) after HIFU ablation of human breast cancer has been investigated. Results show that TILs infiltrated along the margins of the ablated region in all HIFU-treated neoplasms, and the numbers of tumor-infiltrating CD3, CD4, CD8, CD4/CD8, B lymphocytes, and NK cells were increased significantly with HIFU treatment. The number of FasL(+), granzyme(+), and perforin(+) TILs was significantly greater in the HIFU group than in the control group (Fig. 11.10) [69–74].

11.20 Focal, Multifocal, Partial, or HEMI-HIFU Application

Latest treatment options for prostate cancer, which are being considered and already studied, include the development of a precise monofocal or multifocal therapy (25–40 % treatment volume), without TURP (if not obstructed and without strong calcifications or extensive middle lobe) as well as partial therapy (40–90 % treatment volume = contralateral nerve sparing and with TUR).

HEMI-HIFU ablates one single lobe only (<50%); partial (=potency protective or nerve sparing) HIFU excludes a minimum of 5 mm of the contralateral capsule and neurovascular bundle and treats up to 90% of prostatic tissue.

Patients qualifying for one of these approaches should be advised of the risk of tumor recurrence in the untreated area and have to be informed that they cannot expect PSA Nadir levels as in complete or radical therapy and that a "biochemical follow-up by PSA" depends more on PSA velocity than on PSA level.

Fig. 11.10 HIFU application possibilities. (**a**)
Ablatherm®: ventral and
laterally limited. (**b**) Focal.
One®: 3D perfect anatomical
adaption

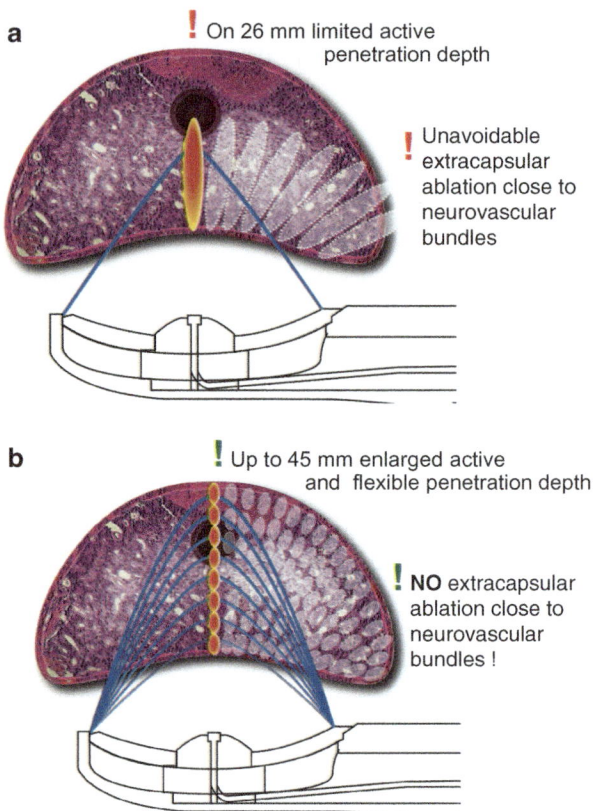

a

! On 26 mm limited active
penetration depth

! Unavoidable
extracapsular
ablation close to
neurovascular
bundles

b

! Up to 45 mm enlarged active
and flexible penetration depth

! **NO** extracapsular
ablation close to
neurovascular
bundles !

A close follow-up of these patients is indispensable. There are several critical issues that need to be addressed regarding focal therapy of prostate cancer: the first of these is the accurate identification and localization of the so-called index lesion within the prostate on which to focus therapy.

> The operator needs to see the tumor and to be sure that there is not tumor if he don't see it.

There are also issues relating to the effectiveness of focal treatments and how patients should be monitored following treatment, whether this is with PSA monitoring, biopsy, or perhaps imaging in the future. These issues are meanwhile stressed sufficiently in three prospective study protocols for focal HIFU recruiting already in the United States, France, and Germany.

> Patients qualifying for focal HIFU ablation should have 1–2 unilateral biopsies Gleason 6, maximum 5 % Gleason 7a, and a PSAi < 10 ng/ml. There should not be a urinary obstruction or calcifications on the tumor-affected lobe.

Localization of tumor within the gland both before and control after treatment is another important issue. The application and the continued development of a variety of imaging and 3D biopsy techniques are likely to provide improvements in the visualization and assessment of HIFU lesions in the near future. With regard to localizing disease, variable sensitivity of magnetic resonance imaging (MRI) has been reported. Functional imaging techniques such as dynamic contrast-enhanced (DCE) MRI, diffusion-weighted imaging (DWI), and magnetic resonance spectroscopic imaging (MRSI) have been evaluated in an attempt to improve the detection and localization of prostate cancer. Results suggest that vascular information from DCE-MRI or DWI MRI combined with metabolic data from MRSI have extremely good potential for improving the accuracy of defining and staging prostate cancer.

In terms of visualization of the efficacy of HIFU treatment, MRI is the gold-standard technique, and the extent of necrosis can be clearly visualized on gadolinium-enhanced T1-weighted images. MRE might also provide a means of assessing the effects of thermal tissue ablation by measuring the mechanical properties of the lesion. HIFU-induced lesions are visible using standard ultrasound, although there are limitations to the accuracy of this approach.

Other ultrasound-based techniques that might prove useful for assessing the extent of HIFU-induced lesions include contrast-enhanced power Doppler and other techniques that characterize the acoustic properties of tissues.

Focal therapy has been compared with whole-gland ablation in a series of 70 patients. Of the 29 patients with unilateral disease, focal therapy involved ablation of the total peripheral zone and a half portion of transitional zone and resulted in a 77 % negative biopsy rate at 12 months. Of the remaining 41 patients with bilateral disease, whole-gland ablation resulted in an 84 % negative biopsy rate at 12 months. Two-year biochemical recurrence-free survival rates were 91 and 50 % for low- and intermediate-risk groups undergoing whole-gland ablation compared with 83 and 54 %, respectively, for the focal therapy equivalents. Morbidity with the two forms of HIFU was comparable [75–80].

Conclusion

PSA was in "Pandora's box" – as Richard J Ablin says – and it is now open!

PSA triggers the diagnosis of PCa detection and it is usually diagnosed earlier than 25 years ago. Patient's life expectancy as well is longer and therefore the diagnostic and therapeutic period is significantly extended. Besides this, resources for medical therapy are not increasing in the same way; new cost-effective noninvasive diagnostics and therapies have to be developed. PCa therapy changes to an individualized, multimodal, sequential therapy, which opens a large space for minimal invasive therapies. Transrectal HIFU for prostate cancer therapy by Ablatherm® is a precise, robotic, evolving, safe, and effective treatment which might fit in this gap.

HIFU allows treatment of the whole spectrum of possible indications in all PCa tumor stages and after all pretreatments, with of course different results and side effects in each indication group. HIFU by Ablatherm® enables to delay or substitute onset of radical classical therapies as radiation, surgery, and ADT by an individualized local, noninvasive tumor ablation in any stage of the disease.

HIFU as a "single-session noninvasive ablation therapy of the endourologist" deserves a different, wider look onto the therapy of prostate cancer: focal therapy and are best samples of the enlarged indication range.

References

1. Fry WJ, Mosberg WH, Barnard JW, et al. Production of focal tissue destructive lesions in the central nervous system with ultrasound. J Neurosurg. 1954;11(5):471–8; PMID 13201985.
2. Ganzer R, Fritsche HM, Brandtner A, Bründl J, Koch D, Wieland WF, Blana A. Fourteen-year oncological and functional outcomes of high-intensity focused ultrasound in localized prostate cancer. BJU Int. 2013;112(3):322–9. doi:10.1111/j.1464-410X.2012.11715.x.
3. Crouzet S, Chapelon JY, Rouvière O, Mege-Lechevallier F, Colombel M, Tonoli-Catez H, Martin X, Gelet A. Whole-gland ablation of localized prostate cancer with high-intensity focused ultrasound: oncologic outcomes and morbidity in 1002 patients. Eur Urol. 2014;65(5):907–14. doi:10.1016/j.eururo.2013.04.039.
4. Thueroff S, Chaussy CG. Evolution and outcomes of 3 MHz high intensity focused ultrasound therapy for localized prostate cancer during 15 years. J Urol. 2013;190(2):702–10. doi:10.1016/j.juro.2013.02.010.
5. Baco E, Blana A, Berge V, Chaussy C, Ganzer R, Crouzet S, Pastizier G, Paulesu Robertson CN, Thueroff S, Wrad JF Sanches-Sala R, Gelet A. Age stratified outcomes after primary HIFU for organ localized prostate cancer in the series of 5206 patients. J Urol. 2013;189(4S) Supplement; abstract 1205:e494. doi:http://dx.doi.org/10.1016/j.juro.2013.02.2559.
6. Uchida T, Nakano M, Hongo S, Shoji S, Nagat Y, Satoh T, Baba S, Usui Y, Terachi T. High intensity ultrasound therapy for prostate cancer. Int J Urol. 2011;19:187–210. doi:10.1111/j1442-2042.2011.02936.x.
7. Lynn JG, Putman TJ. Histological and cerebral lesions produced by focused ultrasound. Am J Pathol. 1944;20(3):637–49. PMC2033152.
8. Ter Haar G. Intervention and therapy. Ultrasound Med Biol. 2000;23(S1):51–4. doi:10.1016/S0301-5629(00)00164-2.
9. Chapelon JY, Margonari J, Theillère Y, Gorry F, Vernier F, Blanc E, Gelet A. Effects of high-energy focused ultrasound on kidney tissue in the rat and the dog. Eur Urol. 1992;22(2):147–52. PMID:1478231.
10. Uchida T, Sanghvi NT, Gardner TA, Koch MO, Ishii D, Minei S, Satoh T, Hyodo Irie A, Baba S. Transrectal high-intensity focused ultrasound for treatment of patients with stage T1b-2n0m0 localized prostate cancer: a preliminary report. Urology. 2002;59(3):394–9. doi:10.1016/S0090-4295(01)01624-7.
11. Chapelon JY, Cathignol D, Cain C, Ebbini E, Kluiwstra JU, Sapozhnikov OA, Fleury G, Berriet R, Chupin L, Guey JL. New piezoelectric transducers for therapeutic ultrasound. Ultrasound Med Biol. 2000;26(1):153–9. doi:10.1016/S0301-5629(99)00120-9.

12. Curiel L, Chavrier F, Souchon R, Birer A, Chapelon JY. 1.5-D high intensity focused ultra-sound array for non-invasive prostate cancer surgery. IEEE Trans Ultrason Ferroelectr Freq Control. 2002;49(2):231–42. doi:10.1109/58.985707.
13. Tan JS, Frizzell LA, Sanghvi N, Wu SJ, Seip R, Kouzmanoff JT. Ultrasound phased arrays for prostate treatment. J Acoust Soc Am. 2001;109(6):3055–64. PMID: 11425148.
14. Damianou CA, Sanghvi NT, Fry FJ. Ultrasonics symposium proceedings. J Acoust Soc Am. 1997;102(1):628–34. doi:10.1109/ULTSYM.1995.495776.
15. Hynynen K, Freund WR, Cline HE, Chung AH, Watkins RD, Vetro JP, Jolesz F. A clinical, noninvasive, MR imaging-monitored ultrasound surgery method. Radiographics. 1996; 16(1):185–95; PMID: 10946699.
16. Damianou C, Pavlou M, Velev O, Kyriakou K. High intensity focused ultrasound ablation of kidney guided by MRI. Ultrasound Med Biol. 2004;30(3):397–404; PMID 15063522.
17. Wu T, Felmlee JP, Greenleaf JF, Riederer SJ, Ehman RL. Assessment of thermal tissue ablation with MR elastography. Magn Reson Med. 2001;45(1):80–7. doi:10.1002/1522-2594(200101)45:1<80::AID-MRM1012>3.0.CO;2-Y.
18. Vaezy S, Shi X, Martin RW, Chi E, Nelson PI, Bailey MR, Crum LA. Real-time visualization of high-intensity focused ultrasound treatment using ultrasound imaging. Ultrasound Med Biol. 2001;27(1):33–42. doi:10.1016/S0301-5629(00)00279-9.
19. Sedelaar JP, Aarnink RP, Van Leenders GJ, Beerlage HP, Debruyne FM, Wijkstra H, De La Rosette JJ. The application of three-dimensional contrast-enhanced ultrasound to measure volume of affected tissue after HIFU treatment for localized prostate cancer. Eur Urol. 2000;37(5):559–68. doi:10.1159/000020193.
20. Yang FY, Teng MC, Lu M, Liang HF, Lee YR, Yen CC, Liang ML, Wong TT. Treating glioblastoma multiforme with selective high dose liposomal doxorubicin chemotherapy induced by repeated focused ultrasound. Int J Nanomedicine. 2012;7:965–74. doi:10.2147/IJN.S29229.
21. Fry FJ, Johnson LK. Tumor irradiation with intense ultrasound. Ultrasound Med Biol. 1978;4(4):337–41. doi:10.1016/0301-5629(78)90022-4.
22. Yang R, Reilly CR, Rescorla FJ, Faught PR, Sanghvi NT, Fry FJ, Franklin Jr TD, Lumeng L, Grosfeld JL. High Intensity focused ultrasound in the treatment of experimental liver cancer. Arch Surg. 1991;126(8):1002–9, discussion 1009–10; PMID: 1863205.
23. Bailey MR, Khokhlova A, Sapozhnikov OA, Kargl SG, Crum LA. Physical mechanism of therapeutic effect of ultrasound (a review). Acoust Phys. 2003;49(4):369–88. doi:10.1134/1.1591291.
24. Chapelon JY, Margonari J, Vernier F, Gorry F, Ecochard R, Gelet A. In vivo effects of high intensity ultrasound on prostatic adenocarcinoma Dunning R3327. Cancer Res. 1992;52: 6353–7; PMID: 1423282.
25. Oosterhof GO, Cornel EB, Smits GA, Debruyne FM, Schalken JA. Influence of high intensity focused ultrasound on the development of metastases. Eur Urol. 1997;32(1):91–5. doi:10.1016/0301-5629(95)02051-9.
26. Adams JB, Moore RG, Anderson JH. High intensity focused ultrasound ablation of rabbit kidney tumors. J Endourol. 1996;10:71–5; PMID 8833733.
27. Köhrmann KU, Michel MS, Steidler A, Marlinghaus E, Kraut O, Alken P. Technical characterization of an ultrasound source for non-invasive thermoablation by high-intensity focused ultrasound. BJU Int. 2002;90(3):248–52; PMID: 12133060.
28. Watkin NA, Morris SB, Rivens IH, Ter Haar GR. High Intensity focused ultrasound ablation of kidney in large animal model. J Endourol. 1997;11(3):191–6; PMID: 9181449.
29. Damianou C. In vitro and in vivo ablation of porcine renal tissue using high intensity focused ultrasound. Ultrasound Med Biol. 2003;29(9):1321–30; PMID: 14553810.
30. Foster RS, Bihrle R, Sanghvi N, Fry F, Kopecky K, Regan J, Eble J, Hennige C, Hennige LV, Donohue JP. Production of prostatic lesions in canines using transrectally administered high intensity focused ultrasound. Eur Urol. 1993;23(2):330–6; PMID: 7683997.
31. Gelet A, Chapelon JY, Margonari J, Theillere Y, Gorry F, Cathignol D, Blanc E. Prostatic tissue destruction by high-intensity focused ultrasound: experimentation on canine prostate. J Endourol. 1993;7(3):249–53. doi:10.1089/end.1993.7.249.

32. Madersbacher S, Pedevilla M, Vingers L, et al. Effect of high intensity focused ultrasound on human prostate cancer in vivo. Cancer Res. 1995;55:3346–51; PMID: 7542168.
33. Madersbacher S, Schatzl G, Djavan B, Stulnig T, Marberger M. Long term outcome of transrectal high intensity focused ultrasound therapy for benign prostate hyperplasia. Eur Urol. 2000;37:687–94; PMID:10828669.
34. Sanghvi NT, et al. High intensity focused ultrasound (HIFU) treatment of BPH: results of multicenter phase III study. Ultrasound Med Biol. 2003;29:S102.
35. Thueroff S, Chaussy CG, Vallancien G, Wieland W, Kiel HJ, Le Duc A, Desgrandchamps F, De La Rosette JJ, Gelet A. High-intensity focused ultrasound and localized prostate cancer: efficacy results from the European Multicentric Study. J Endourol. 2003;17(8):673–7. doi:10.1089/089277903322518699.
36. Rebillard X, Davin JL, Soulié M, Comité de Cancérologie de l'Association Française d'Urologie. Treatment by HIFU of prostate cancer: survey of literature and treatment indications. Prog Urol. 2003;13(6):1428–56; PMID: 15000326.
37. Vallancien G, Prapotnich D, Cathelineau X, Baumert H, Rozet F. Transrectal focused ultrasound combined with transurethral resection of the prostate for the treatment of localized prostate cancer: feasibility study. J Urol. 2004;171(6):2265–7; PMID 15126799.
38. Chaussy CG, Thueroff S. The status of high-intensity focused ultrasound in the treatment of localized prostate cancer and the impact of a combined resection. Curr Urol Rep. 2003;4(3):248–52; PMID: 12756090.
39. Beerlage HP, Van Leenders GJ, Oosterhof GO, Witjes JA, Ruijter ET, Van de Kaa CA, Debruyne FM, De la Rosette JJ. High-intensity focused ultrasound (HIFU) followed after one to two weeks by radical retropubic prostatectomy: results of a prospective study. Prostate. 1999;39(1):41–6; PMID: 10221265.
40. Rouviere O, Lyonnet D, Raudrant A, Colin-Pangaud C, Chapelon JY, Bouvier R, Dubernard JM, Gelet A. MRI appearance of prostate following transrectal HIFU ablation of localized cancer. Eur Urol. 2001;40(3):265–74; PMID: 11684842.
41. D'Amico AV, Moul J, Carroll PR, Sun L, Lubeck D, Chen MH. Cancer-specific mortality after surgery or radiation for patients with clinically localized prostate cancer managed during the prostate specific antigen era. J Clin Oncol. 2003;21(11):2163–72; PMID: 12775742.
42. Ganzer R, Rogenhofer S, Walter B, Lunz JC, Schostak M, Wieland WF, Blana A. PSA nadir is a significant predictor of treatment failure after high-intensity focused ultrasound (HIFU) treatment of localized prostate cancer. Eur Urol. 2008;53(3):547–53; PMID: 17662520.
43. Ganzer R, Robertson CN, Ward JF, Brown SC, Conti GN, Murat FJ, Pasticier G, Rebillard X, Thueroff S, Wieland WF, Blana A. Correlation of prostate-specific antigen Nadir and biochemical failure after High-Intensity Focused Ultrasound of localized prostate cancer based on the Stuttgart failure criteria – analysis from the @-Registry. BJU Int. 2011;108(8 Pt 2):E196–201; PMID: 21332907.
44. Pinthus JH, Farrokhyar F, Hassouna MM, Woods E, Whelan K, Shayegan B, Orovan WL. Single session primary high-intensity focused ultrasonography treatment of localized prostate cancer: biochemical outcomes during third generation-based technology. BJU Int. 2012;110(8):1142–8; PMID 22372721.
45. Blana A, Murat FJ, Walter B, Thueroff S, Wieland WF, Chaussy CG, Gelet A. First analysis of the long-term results with transrectal HIFU in patients with localised prostate cancer. Eur Urol. 2008;53(6):1194–201; PMID: 17997026.
46. Chaussy CG, Thueroff S. Results and side effects of high intensity focused ultrasound in localized prostate cancer. J Endourol. 2001;15(4):437–40, 447–8; PMID 11394458.
47. Gelet A, Chapelon JY, Bouvier R, Rouvière O, Lyonnet D, Dubernard JM. Transrectal high intensity focused ultrasound for the treatment of localized prostate cancer: factors influencing the outcome. Eur Urol. 2001;40(2):124–9; PMID: 11528187.
48. Blana A, Walter B, Rogenhofer S, Wieland WF. High intensity focused ultrasound for the treatment of localized prostate cancer: 5-year experience. Urology. 2004;63(2):297–300; PMID 14972475.

49. Ficarra V, Antoniolli SZ, Novara G, Parisi A, Fra-Calanza S, Martignoni G, Artibani W. Short-term outcome after high-intensity focused ultrasound in the treatment of patients with high-risk prostate cancer. BJU Int. 2006;98(6):1193–8; PMID: 17125477.
50. Poissonnier L, Chapelon JY, Rouvière O, Curiel L, Bouvier R, Martin X, Dubernard JM, Gelet A. Control of prostate cancer by transrectal HIFU in 227 patients. Eur Urol. 2007;51(2):381–7; PMID: 16857310.
51. Blana A, Hierl J, Rogenhofer S, Lunz JC, Wieland WF, Walter B, Ganzer R. Factors predicting for formation of bladder outlet obstruction after high intensity focused ultrasound in treatment of localized prostate cancer. Urology. 2008;71(5):863–7; PMID: 18313119.
52. Thueroff SS. Das inzidentelle Prostatakarzinom im Stadium T1a: Wait and See oder radikale Prostatektomie? Inaugural dissertation, Johannes Gutenberg Universität Mainz; 2009.
53. Thueroff S, Chaussy CG. Therapeutic robotic transrectal ultrasound ablation of incidental prostate cancer after transurethral prostate resection: a prospective single center Pilot Study. Poster 28 presented at EUROSON, Madrid; 2012.
54. Thueroff S, Conti G, Paulesu A, Chaussy CG, Ganzer R, Berge V, Blana A, Baco E, Pasticier G, Crouzet S, Robertson C, Ward J, Gelet A. High intensity focused ultrasound in localized prostate cancer retreatment rate development. Poster 4562 presented at AUA, Orlando; 2014.
55. Thueroff S, Chaussy C. Prostate cancer treatment costs: what influences them? Poster 1036 presented at EAU, Paris; 2006.
56. Netsch C, Bach T, Gross E, Gross AJ. Rectourethral fistula after high intensity focused ultrasound therapy for prostate cancer and its surgical management. Urology. 2011;77(4):999–1004; PMID: 21215427.
57. Fiaschetti V, Manenti G, Di Poce I, Formari M, Rcci A, Finazzo Agrò E, Simonetti G. A recto-urethral fistula due to transrectal high intensity focused ultrasound treatment: diagnosis and management. Case Rep Radiol. 2012. Article ID 962090 http://dx.doi.org/10.1155/2012/962090.
58. Ahmed HU, Ishaq A, Zacharakis E, et al. Rectal fistula after salvage high intensity focused ultrasound for recurrent prostate cancer after combined brachytherapy and external beam radiotherapy. BJU Int. 2009;102:321–3.
59. Chaussy C, Thueroff S. Gleason rise in recurrent prostate cancer after previous prostate cancer therapies? Urology. 2009;74(S4):S214. doi:10.1016/j.urology.2009.07.587.
60. Thueroff S, Chaussy C. Prostate cancer progression under long-term ADT, treated by robotic high intensity focused ultrasound: 10 years efficacy. Poster 1.499 presented at SUI, Berlin; 2001.
61. Uchida T, Shoji S, Nakano M, Hongo S, Nitta M, Usui Y, Nagata Y. High intensity focused ultrasound as salvage therapy for patients with recurrent prostate cancer after external beam radiation, brachytherapy or proton therapy. BJU Int. 2011;107(3):378–82; PMID 21265984.
62. Murato-Kawano A, Nakano M, Hongo S, Shoji S, Nagata Y, Uchida T. Salvage high intensity focused ultrasound for biopsy confirmed local recurrence of prostate cancer after radical prostatectomy. BJU Int. 2010;105:1642–5; PMID: 19922544.
63. Hayashi M, Shinmei S, Asano K. Transrectal high intensity focused ultrasound for treatment for patients with biochemical failure after radical prostatectomy. Int J Urol. 2007;14(11):1048–50; PMID: 17956536.
64. Gelet A, Chapelon JY, Poissonniere L, Bouvier R, Pouviere O, Curiel L, Janier M, Vallencien G. Local recurrence of prostate cancer after external beam radiotherapy: early experience of salvage therapy using high intensity focused ultrasonography. Urology. 2004;63:625–9; PMID 15072864.
65. Murat FJ, Poissonnier L, Rabilloud M, Belot A, Bouvier R, Rouviere O, Chapelon JY, Gelet A. Mid-term results demonstrate salvage high-intensity focused ultrasound (HIFU) as an effective and acceptably morbid salvage treatment option for locally radiorecurrent prostate cancer. Eur Urol. 2009;55(3):640–7; PMID: 18508188.
66. Chaussy CG, Thueroff S, Bergsdorf T. Local recurrence of prostate cancer after curative therapy. HIFU (Ablatherm) as a treatment option. Urologe A. 2006;45(10):1271–5; PMID 17006697.

67. Berge V, Baco E, Karlsen SJ. A prospective study of salvage high intensity focused ultrasound for locally radiorecurrent prostate cancer: early results. Scan J Urol Nephrol. 2010;44(4):223–7; PMID: 20350272.
68. Chalasani V, Martinez CH, Lim D, Chin J. Salvage HIFU for recurrent prostate cancer after radiotherapy. Prostate Cancer Prostatic Dis. 2008;12:124–9; PMID: 18852702.
69. Xia JZ, Xie FL, Ran FL, Xie XP, Fan YM, Wu F. High intensity focused ultrasound tumor ablation activates autologous tumor specific cytotoxic T-lymphocytes. Ultrasound Med Biol. 2012;38(8):1363–71; PMID 22633269.
70. Huang X, Yuan F, Liang M, Lo HW, Shinohara ML, Robertson C, Zhong P. M-HIFU inhibits tumour growth, suppresses STAT3 activity and enhances tumour specific immunity in a transplant tumor model of prostate cancer. PLoS One. 2012;7(7):e41632; PMID: 22911830.
71. Kiel HJ, Thueroff S, Laumer M, Heymann J, Chaussy C, Mackensen A. Indication of systemic PSA specific T-cell responses in prostate cancer patients after high-intensity focused ultrasound treatment. Poster 317 presented at EAU Congress 2005 in Istanbul. Eur Urol Suppl. 2005;4(3):53. doi:10.1016/S1569-9056(05)80211-8.
72. Lu P, Zhu XQ, Xu ZL, Zhou Q, Wu F. Increased infiltration of activated tumor infiltrating lymphocytes after high intensity focused ultrasound ablation of human breast cancer. Surgery. 2009;145(3):286–93; PMID: 19231581.
73. Wu F, Wang ZB, Cao YD, Zhou Q, Zhang Y, Xu ZL, Zhu XQ. Expression of tumor antigens and heat-shock protein 70 in breast cancer cells after high intensity focused ultrasound ablation. Ann Surg Oncol. 2007;14(3):1237–42; PMID: 17187168.
74. Wu F, Wang ZB, Lu P, Xu ZL, Chen WC, Zhu H, Jin CB. Activated anti-tumor immunity in cancer patients after high intensity focused ultrasound ablation. Ultrasound Med Biol. 2004;30(9):1217–22; PMID: 15550325.
75. Ahmed HU, Hindley RG, Dickinson L, Freeman A, Kirkham AP, Sahu M, Scott R, Allen C, Van der Meulen J, Emberton M. Focal therapy for localised unifocal and multifocal prostate cancer: a prospective development study. Lancet Oncol. 2012;13(6):622–32; PMID: 22512844.
76. Ahmed HU, Chatcart P, McCartan M, Kirkham A, Allen C, Freeman A, Emberton M. Focal salvage therapy for localized prostate cancer recurrence after external beam radiotherapy: a pilot study. Cancer. 2012;118(17):4148–55; PMID: 22907704.
77. Crouzet S, Rouviere O, Martin X, Gelet A. High intensity focused ultrasound as focal therapy of prostate cancer. Curr Opin Urol. 2014;24(3):225–30; PMID: 24710053.
78. Muto S, Yoshii T, Saito K, Kamijama Y, Die H, Horie S. Focal therapy with high-intensity-focused ultrasound in the treatment of localized prostate cancer. Jpn J Clin Oncol. 2008;38(3):192–9; PMID: 18281309.
79. El Fegoun AB, Baret E, Prapotnich D, Soon S, Cathelineau X, Rozet F, Galinao M, Sanhcez-Salaz R, Vallencien G. Focal therapy with high-intensity focused ultrasound for prostate cancer in elderly. A feasibility study with 10 years follow-up. Int Braz J Urol. 2011;37(2):213–9; discussion 220–2; PMID 21557838.
80. Nomura T, Mimata H. Focal therapy in the management f prostate cancer. An emerging approach for localized prostate cancer. Adv Urol. 2012;(2012):article ID 391437; PMID: 22593764.
81. Baco E, Gelet A, Crouzet S, Rud E, Rouvière O, Tonoli-Catez H, Berge V, Chapelon JY, Eggesbø HB. Hemi salvage high-intensity focused ultrasound (HIFU) in unilateral radiorecurrent prostate cancer: a prospective two-centre study. BJU Int Urol Oncol. 2014. doi:10.1111/bju.12545.
82. Chaussy CG, Tilki D, Thueroff S. Transrectal high intensity focused ultrasound for the treatment of localized prostate cancer: current role. JCT. 2013;4(4A):59–73. doi:10.4236/jct.2013.44A007.
83. Guimaraes GC, De Cassio Zequi S, Thueroff S. Chapter.113. Terapias fisicas, ablativa e tratamentos focais para Cancer de prostata. In: Borges Dos Reis R, De Cassio Zequi S, Zertai M, editors. Urologia moderna. Societa Brasiliana d'Urologia; 2014. p. 1001–7.
84. Thueroff S, Herzog K, Chaussy CG, Solovov Y, Dvoinikov S, Vozdvizhenskiy M. Effect of intensified training on learning curve for robotic high intensity focused ultrasound (rHIFU) in advanced

prostate cancer therapy. Urology: Gold Journal" and official publisher of SIU. 2009;74(S4):S134. doi:10.1016/j.urology.2009.07.1346.

85. Chaussy C, Thueroff S. Recto-urethral fistulae formation after transrectal pulsed high intensity focused ultrasound (HIFU). Poster presented at 23rd EAU congress. Eur Urol Suppl. 2008;7(3):118. doi:10.1016/S1569-9056(08)60191-8.

86. Shaplysin LV, Solov VA, Vosdvizhenskiï MO, Khametov RZ. High-intensity focused ultrasound (HIFU) for the prostate cancer treatment: 5-year results. Urology. 2013;1:70–2 (Russian) PMID: 23662500.

Future Uro-technologies: Hope or Hell for Prostate Cancer Patients?

12

Alexandre Ingels, M. Pilar Laguna,
and Jean J.M.C.H. de la Rosette

Contents

12.1   Introduction

The concept of focal therapy first rose up with lumpectomy for breast cancer. The preservation of healthy glands surrounding the tumor allowed to minimize esthetic damage with its psychological impact on women and remained safe in terms of oncologic outcomes, as far as resection margins around the tumor had been respected [1]. Secondly, partial nephrectomy for small renal masses with surgical excision of the tumor, sparing ipsilateral nephrons, proved to be also an oncologically safe

A. Ingels • M.P. Laguna • J.J.M.C.H. de la Rosette (✉)
Department of Urology, Academisch Medisch Centrum,
Postbus 22660, Amsterdam 1100DD, The Netherlands
e-mail: Alexandre.ingels@gmail.com; j.j.delarosette@amc.uva.nl

© Springer International Publishing Switzerland 2015
S. Thüroff, C.G. Chaussy (eds.), *Focal Therapy of Prostate Cancer:
An Emerging Strategy for Minimally Invasive, Staged Treatment*,
DOI 10.1007/978-3-319-14160-2_12

procedure with longtime preservation of kidney function and prevention of cardio-vascular death compared to radical nephrectomy [2, 3]. Equivalent strategies exist for the thyroid [4], liver [5, 6], and pancreas (Whipple procedure) [7]. This paradigm should be extended to prostate cancer where tissue preservation in this situation would not lead to esthetic or overall survival gain but to quality of life improvement mostly due to urinary, sexual, and intestinal side effects of whole-mount gland ablation. The challenging localization of the prostate into the pelvis and its anatomical relations with functional or dangerous structures such as the urethral sphincter, rectum, neurovascular bundles, and dorsal venous complex make its surgical partial ablation hardly conceivable, and no such series had been reported to our knowledge. From this statement, new uro-technologies appear as a no-brainer to face this challenge. Many new ablative technologies seem to offer an alternative between a functionally mutilating radical treatment (radical prostatectomy or external beam radiation therapy) and a potentially undertreating active surveillance. To date, there is no randomized controlled trial comparing focal technique to another or focal technique to radical treatment and/or active surveillance. As a result, most of the practices are based on a lower level of evidence. Although the use of this new oncological approach for small prostate cancer starts to spread throughout the urological community, supported by encouraging clinical outcomes, some caveat have to be emphasized in order to prevent this new hope for patient management in terms of functional outcomes from turning to hell.

12.2 Hope of Focal Therapy

12.2.1 Minimally Invasive Techniques for Small Tumors

Numerous ablative techniques had been developed by industries during the last decade and described in previous chapters of this book: cryosurgery, high-intensity focal ultrasound (HIFU), photodynamic therapy (PDT), laser therapy, brachytherapy, irreversible electroporation (IRE), etc. All of them use either transrectal (HIFU) or transperineal percutaneous needle approaches (cryotherapy, IRE, brachytherapy, laser therapy, PDT, radiofrequency ablation). There are also different tissue-preserving strategies used across different series: hockey stick, hemiablation, multifocal, and unifocal [8]. All these techniques and strategies aimed to be less invasive than radical treatment in terms of surgical approach but also in terms of functional tissue preservation: neurobundles to preserve potency, urethral sphincter to preserve continence, and Denonvilliers fascia to prevent rectal toxicity. The length of hospital stay is often considered as a surrogate to measure the efficacy of a less invasive surgical technique. In their recent review, Valerio et al. analyzed data from 25 studies reporting focal therapy for prostate cancer in the primary setting. Among 14 series reporting on the length of hospital stay, the overall median length was 1 day. In a less recent study, Lotan et al. compared the length of hospital stay for patients undergoing radical prostatectomy with retropubic, laparoscopic, or robot-assisted approaches in order to assess overall cost of the three techniques. The mean length of hospital stay was respectively of 2.5, 1.3, and 1.2 days [9]. Although those results should be interpreted with caution (the length of hospital stay is very dependent on the healthcare system of each country), they give us a general idea and fit with our common sense that needle surgery is probably less invasive than open, laparoscopic, or robot-assisted surgery.

Another way to estimate the invasiveness of a technique is to control the quality of life before and after the procedure. In their review, Valerio et al. [8] reported urinary functional outcomes using validated questionnaires from nine studies; the pad-free continence rate varied between 95 and 100 %, and the range of leak-free rates was 83–100 %. Erectile function was reported using validated questionnaires in 10 studies. Erectile function sufficient for penetration was reported in 54–100 % of patients (with or without PDE5-I medication). Rectal toxicity was often poorly reported. When it was reported, rates of fistula ranged from 0 to 1 %. In a prospectively designed study, Sanda et al. compared quality of life outcomes after primary treatment of prostate cancer using the three main whole-mount gland treatment strategies: radical prostatectomy, external beam radiation therapy, or brachytherapy. The percentage of patients reporting no problem or small problems for sexual function, urinary continence, and bowel/rectal function using a self-questionnaire was, respectively, 50, 92, and 98 % for patients treated by radical prostatectomies; 69, 95, and 89 % for radiotherapies; and 70, 95, and 91 % for brachytherapies [10]. Although only randomized controlled trials could bring a definitive statement on this topic, focal therapy seems to fulfill the main aim to be less invasive than radical treatments.

12.2.2 Treatment of Radiation Failure

Another promising application of focal therapy is the treatment of local recurrence after external beam radiation therapy (EBRT) for prostate cancer. The overall local relapse rate after EBRT is estimated to be around 30 % on prostate biopsies performed at least 2 years after EBRT [11–13]. This recurrence rate is significantly lower with high-dose radiation compared with conventional doses. Most men presenting cancer relapse after EBRT are treated with androgen deprivation therapies, a systemic strategy involving serious impacts on the quality of life and cardiac, bone, and metabolic health [14, 15]. Most patients presenting a local recurrence are suitable for a local salvage treatment. Several whole-mount prostate treatments have been explored with acceptable oncological results [16–18]: radical prostatectomy, cryoablation, HIFU, and brachytherapy. When used in already irradiated tissue, these techniques present higher rates of genitourinary and bowel morbidity than for primary settings because of the previous damages of the surrounding structures. Approximately 66 % of men who have localized failure after EBRT can develop recurrent unifocal or unilateral cancer, and the main site of recurrence is usually the site of the index lesion before primary treatment [19–23]. From this statement, the rationale of focal salvage therapy would be to target this zone with safety margins in order to spare noncancerous tissue and respect the surrounding structures. Several studies have reported the feasibility of focal salvage therapy using brachytherapy

[24], cryoablation [25–27], HIFU [28], or radiofrequency interstitial tumor ablation (RITA) [29]. From oncological perspectives, those studies reported positive biopsy rates ranging from 8 to 10 % when using TRUS biopsies and 44 % when using transperineal template mapping biopsies for a median range follow-up of 17–47 months [8]; only one series reported the presence of residual significant cancer with a rate of 8 % [27]. The overall survival was 100 % in the two series that reported this outcome [27, 29]. Focal salvage treatment functional outcomes can hardly be generalized from the limited data available in literature. Continence, estimated by the pad-free rate, was achieved in 87.2–100 % of patients. In three studies ($n=82$), potency was preserved in 29–40 % of previously potent patients [25, 27, 28]. The rate of rectourethral fistula (0–12 %) was significantly higher than in the primary cases [8]. Although the number of patients included was limited and a large randomized controlled trial to validate this strategy is still awaited, all these studies concluded in the feasibility of focal therapy in the frame of local recurrence post-radiotherapy. It seems to be a pertinent option when patients are properly selected.

12.2.3 Re-treatment Without Problems

Finally, another advantage of focal therapy, although it is hardly demonstrated in literature, is the possibility to treat and re-treat safely the prostate with the same technique. Twelve series reported the need for secondary focal treatments with a range of 0–34 % [8]; this re-treatment is feasible and allows another chance to preserve genitourinary and bowel functions to the patients or, in the case of a second relapse, to postpone radical treatment and associated side effects.

12.3   How Hope Could Turn to Hell

12.3.1 Uncertainty If All Cancer Is Gone

One limitation of focal therapy is the absence of a surgical specimen to analyze in order to check the procedure quality. Just like EBRT, this statement has two negative consequences to deal with: first is the uncertainty if all cancer is gone. Did ablative margins safely enclose the whole tumor? Had all central tumor cells been ablated efficiently? Second is the inability to confirm imaging- and biopsy-based tumor grading and staging. It has been shown that tumor upgrading and upstaging occur in respectively 6–36 % [30–32] and 27–57 % [33] from biopsy and imaging to surgical specimen analysis. Patients treated with radical prostatectomy can benefit from this pathological control by being potentially reclassified in a worse-prognosis risk group and receiving adjuvant treatment to improve their survival. This limitation has to be compensated by a thorough follow-up based on control biopsy, preferably transperineal template mapping biopsies (TTMB), never as sensitive as whole-mount prostate section analysis, and accurate imaging strategy including multiparametric MRI.

12.3.2 Metastasis Development

Another challenge of focal therapy is the follow-up based on poorly known consequences of this new strategy on the disease natural history. Cancer relapse is well
defined in the frame of whole-mount prostate treatment (prostatectomy or EBRT):
clinical evidence of recurrence, 2 consecutive PSA values of 0.2 ng/mL or greater
after radical prostatectomy, and rise of 2 ng/mL above the posttreatment PSA nadir
after radiation therapy [34]. Focal therapy does not have such a well-defined, validated PSA cut point to define biochemical failure. It is hard to assess how much
healthy gland has been spared during the procedure and how far this remaining
prostate tissue is responsible for posttreatment PSA level. An important prognosis
marker for prostate cancer is PSA velocity or PSA doubling time, often used to
choose therapeutic options after post-curative treatment biochemical failure. The
calculation of PSA doubling time is based on the assumption that PSA follows an
exponential pattern in case of relapse. To our knowledge, this statement has never
been confirmed after focal therapy. We do not know if PSA doubling time can be
used as a prognostic marker and what would be a sensitive cutoff to search for local
or systemic recurrence. There is still a broad field of research to understand how the
cancer behaves in case of relapse and what would be pertinent markers to trigger
specific diagnostic investigations to search for local or metastatic progression.

12.3.3 Development of Significant Complications Such as Fistula and Incontinence

With focal therapy being a recent strategy, competing on one side with active surveillance and on the other side with radical treatments, there are still improvements
to be made to better select candidates and to standardize what zone to ablate and
with which energy. Although functional outcomes seem promising, there are still
cases of rectourethral fistula [35] and incontinence reported [8]. As a minimally
invasive technique, those side effects should be exceptional and could probably be
reduced by standardization of techniques and definition of criteria predicting those
side effects, allowing a better hazard control.

12.3.4 New Technologies Without Standing the Test of Time

The most important danger of focal therapy is inherent with the development of new
technologies encouraging the rapid spread of new techniques, shortcutting the real
bottleneck of medical innovation validation: the randomized controlled trial. There is
a time frame to seize the opportunity of a clinical trial for new surgical technologies,
between safety validation on preclinical models and the empirical adoption of this
new technique by a large surgeon community that would make it hard to compare
new techniques with the original standard one. The classical example to illustrate this
fact is the development of robot-assisted radical prostatectomy (RARP): no

prospective randomized controlled trial had been led to compare it with open radical or laparoscopic prostatectomies in order to obtain approval of this technique. Today we probably missed the train, and it is very unlikely that a large prospective trial can be designed with clinicians and patients accepting to be included in the controlled arm of open prostatectomy while they could benefit the pretended better technique of RARP. This problem of safe and rigorous evaluation is particularly challenging for surgical techniques compared to new drug development since it requires good collaborations inside surgeons' community.

Conclusion

To conclude, we have reasons to be optimistic and should encourage the development of focal therapy for prostate cancer. Although pertinent evidences are still lacking, it seems to be a minimally invasive technique allowing shorter hospital stay and less complications while remaining a safe curative treatment. There is certainly a place for focal therapy as a salvage treatment after external beam radiation treatment failure, and we hope to see this technique as a safe way to re-treat cancer and preserve genitourinary and bowel functions better than current mutilating whole-mount gland treatments. As a minimally invasive treatment, most of the focal techniques allow re-treatment of the gland after evidences of first treatment failure (positive biopsy for significant residual cancer).

Our enthusiasm should not blind us from potential hazards associated with focal therapy. The inability to control the prostate after treatment because of the absence of pathological specimen should be compensated by standardized and validated follow-up protocols based on accurate imaging (multiparametric MRI) and biopsies. We also need to validate good markers for recurrence detection in the posttreatment follow-up. The significant number of serious complications such as rectourethral fistula or incontinence reported in literature reveals that there are still technical improvements to be made and better patient selection. We believe that the time for proof-of-concept studies is about to be achieved, but the urologist community should not be satisfied by this level of evidence. Now is certainly the right time to launch a prospective controlled trial to validate the different focal therapy techniques and compare them to each other and with active surveillance or radical treatments. This validation requires high-level collaborative works inside urologists' community but also with radiologists, radiotherapists, and pathologists. This effort has to be launched now since we have observed in the past that the time period to conduct such controlled trial for new technologies is limited.

References

1. Fisher B, Anderson S, Bryant J, Margolese RG, Deutsch M, Fisher ER, et al. Twenty-year follow-up of a randomized trial comparing total mastectomy, lumpectomy, and lumpectomy plus irradiation for the treatment of invasive breast cancer. N Engl J Med. 2002;347(16):1233–41.
2. Fergany AF, Hafez KS, Novick AC. Long-term results of nephron sparing surgery for localized renal cell carcinoma: 10-year follow-up. J Urol. 2000;163(2):442–5.

3. Huang WC, Elkin EB, Levey AS, Jang TL, Russo P. Partial nephrectomy versus radical nephrectomy in patients with small renal tumors–is there a difference in mortality and cardiovascular outcomes? J Urol. 2009;181(1):55–61; discussion 61–2.

4. Solomon BL, Wartofsky L, Burman KD. Current trends in the management of well differentiated papillary thyroid carcinoma. J Clin Endocrinol Metab. 1996;81(1):333–9.

5. Kennedy JE, Wu F, ter Haar GR, Gleeson FV, Phillips RR, Middleton MR, et al. High-intensity focused ultrasound for the treatment of liver tumours. Ultrasonics. 2004;42(1–9):931–5.

6. Lencioni R, Cioni D, Crocetti L, Franchini C, Pina CD, Lera J, et al. Early-stage hepatocellular carcinoma in patients with cirrhosis: long-term results of percutaneous image-guided radiofrequency ablation. Radiology. 2005;234(3):961–7.

7. Yeo CJ, Cameron JL, Sohn TA, Lillemoe KD, Pitt HA, Talamini MA, et al. Six hundred fifty consecutive pancreaticoduodenectomies in the 1990s: pathology, complications, and outcomes. Ann Surg. 1997;226(3):248–57; discussion 257–60.

8. Valerio M, Ahmed HU, Emberton M, Lawrentschuk N, Lazzeri M, Montironi R, et al. The role of focal therapy in the management of localised prostate cancer: a systematic review. Eur Urol. 2014;66:732–51.

9. Lotan Y, Cadeddu JA, Gettman MT. The new economics of radical prostatectomy: cost comparison of open, laparoscopic and robot assisted techniques. J Urol. 2004;172(4 Pt 1):1431–5.

10. Sanda MG, Dunn RL, Michalski J, Sandler HM, Northouse L, Hembroff L, et al. Quality of life and satisfaction with outcome among prostate-cancer survivors. N Engl J Med. 2008;358(12):1250–61.

11. Crook J, Malone S, Perry G, Bahadur Y, Robertson S, Abdolell M. Postradiotherapy prostate biopsies: what do they really mean? Results for 498 patients. Int J Radiat Oncol Biol Phys. 2000;48(2):355–67.

12. Pollack A, Zagars GK, Antolak JA, Kuban DA, Rosen II. Prostate biopsy status and PSA nadir level as early surrogates for treatment failure: analysis of a prostate cancer randomized radiation dose escalation trial. Int J Radiat Oncol Biol Phys. 2002;54(3):677–85.

13. Zelefsky MJ, Fuks Z, Hunt M, Lee HJ, Lombardi D, Ling CC, et al. High dose radiation delivered by intensity modulated conformal radiotherapy improves the outcome of localized prostate cancer. J Urol. 2001;166(3):876–81.

14. Grossfeld GD, Li Y-P, Lubeck DP, Broering JM, Mehta SS, Carroll PR. Predictors of secondary cancer treatment in patients receiving local therapy for prostate cancer: data from cancer of the prostate strategic urologic research endeavor. J Urol. 2002;168(2):530–5.

15. Taylor LG, Canfield SE, Du XL. Review of major adverse effects of androgen-deprivation therapy in men with prostate cancer. Cancer. 2009;115(11):2388–99.

16. Nguyen PL, D'Amico AV, Lee AK, Suh WW. Patient selection, cancer control, and complications after salvage local therapy for postradiation prostate-specific antigen failure: a systematic review of the literature. Cancer. 2007;110(7):1417–28.

17. Boukaram C, Hannoun-Levi J-M. Management of prostate cancer recurrence after definitive radiation therapy. Cancer Treat Rev. 2010;36(2):91–100.

18. Zacharakis E, Ahmed HU, Ishaq A, Scott R, Illing R, Freeman A, et al. The feasibility and safety of high-intensity focused ultrasound as salvage therapy for recurrent prostate cancer following external beam radiotherapy. BJU Int. 2008;102(7):786–92.

19. Huang WC, Kuroiwa K, Serio AM, Bianco Jr FJ, Fine SW, Shayegan B, et al. The anatomical and pathological characteristics of irradiated prostate cancers may influence the oncological efficacy of salvage ablative therapies. J Urol. 2007;177(4):1324–9; quiz 1591.

20. Pucar D, Hricak H, Shukla-Dave A, Kuroiwa K, Drobnjak M, Eastham J, et al. Clinically significant prostate cancer local recurrence after radiation therapy occurs at the site of primary tumor: magnetic resonance imaging and step-section pathology evidence. Int J Radiat Oncol Biol Phys. 2007;69(1):62–9.

21. Cellini N, Morganti AG, Mattiucci GC, Valentini V, Leone M, Luzi S, et al. Analysis of intraprostatic failures in patients treated with hormonal therapy and radiotherapy: implications for conformal therapy planning. Int J Radiat Oncol Biol Phys. 2002;53(3):595–9.

22. Arakawa A, Song S, Scardino PT, Wheeler TM. High grade prostatic intraepithelial neoplasia in prostates removed following irradiation failure in the treatment of prostatic adenocarcinoma. Pathol Res Pract. 1995;191(9):868–72.
23. Cheng L, Cheville JC, Pisansky TM, Sebo TJ, Slezak J, Bergstralh EJ, et al. Prevalence and distribution of prostatic intraepithelial neoplasia in salvage radical prostatectomy specimens after radiation therapy. Am J Surg Pathol. 1999;23(7):803–8.
24. Nguyen PL, Chen M-H, D'Amico AV, Tempany CM, Steele GS, Albert M, et al. Magnetic resonance image-guided salvage brachytherapy after radiation in select men who initially presented with favorable-risk prostate cancer: a prospective phase 2 study. Cancer. 2007;110(7):1485–92.
25. Eisenberg ML, Shinohara K. Partial salvage cryoablation of the prostate for recurrent prostate cancer after radiotherapy failure. Urology. 2008;72(6):1315–8.
26. Gowardhan B, Greene D. Salvage cryotherapy: is there a role for focal therapy? J Endourol. 2010;24(5):861–4.
27. De Castro Abreu AL, Bahn D, Leslie S, Shoji S, Silverman P, Desai MM, et al. Salvage focal and salvage total cryoablation for locally recurrent prostate cancer after primary radiation therapy. BJU Int. 2013;112(3):298–307.
28. Ahmed HU, Cathcart P, McCartan N, Kirkham A, Allen C, Freeman A, et al. Focal salvage therapy for localized prostate cancer recurrence after external beam radiotherapy: a pilot study. Cancer. 2012;118(17):4148–55.
29. Shariat SF, Raptidis G, Masatoschi M, Bergamaschi F, Slawin KM. Pilot study of radiofrequency interstitial tumor ablation (RITA) for the treatment of radio-recurrent prostate cancer. Prostate. 2005;65(3):260–7.
30. Cohen MS, Hanley RS, Kurteva T, Ruthazer R, Silverman ML, Sorcini A, et al. Comparing the Gleason prostate biopsy and Gleason prostatectomy grading system: the Lahey Clinic Medical Center experience and an international meta-analysis. Eur Urol. 2008;54(2):371–81.
31. Kuroiwa K, Shiraishi T, Naito S, Clinicopathological Research Group for Localized Prostate Cancer Investigators. Gleason score correlation between biopsy and prostatectomy specimens and prediction of high-grade Gleason patterns: significance of central pathologic review. Urology. 2011;77(2):407–11.
32. Djavan B, Kadesky K, Klopukh B, Marberger M, Roehrborn CG. Gleason scores from prostate biopsies obtained with 18-gauge biopsy needles poorly predict Gleason scores of radical prostatectomy specimens. Eur Urol. 1998;33(3):261–70.
33. Gleason DF. Undergrading of prostate cancer biopsies: a paradox inherent in all biologic bivariate distributions. Urology. 1996;47(3):289–91.
34. Heidenreich A, Bastian PJ, Bellmunt J, Bolla M, Joniau S, van der Kwast T, et al. EAU guidelines on prostate cancer. Part 1: screening, diagnosis, and local treatment with curative intent-update 2013. Eur Urol. 2014;65(1):124–37.
35. Ahmed HU, Freeman A, Kirkham A, Sahu M, Scott R, Allen C, et al. Focal therapy for localized prostate cancer: a phase I/II trial. J Urol. 2011;185(4):1246–54.

Index

© Springer International Publishing Switzerland 2015
S. Thüroff, C.G. Chaussy (eds.), *Focal Therapy of Prostate Cancer:*
An Emerging Strategy for Minimally Invasive, Staged Treatment,
DOI 10.1007/978-3-319-14160-2

GPSR Compliance

The European Union's (EU) General Product Safety Regulation (GPSR)
is a set of rules that requires consumer products to be safe and our
obligations to ensure this.

If you have any concerns about our products, you can contact us on
ProductSafety@springernature.com

In case Publisher is established outside the EU, the EU authorized
representative is:

Springer Nature Customer Service Center GmbH
Europaplatz 3
69115 Heidelberg, Germany

Batch number: 09636403

Printed by Printforce, the Netherlands